THINK
HEALTHY
CHOOSE
HEALTHY

MAKE HEALTHIER DIETARY AND LIFESTYLE
CHOICES THROUGH THE HOLISTIC APPROACH
OF NUTRITION AND AYURVEDA

VARSHA KHATRI

Varsha Khatri

BALBOA.PRESS
A DIVISION OF HAY HOUSE

Balboa Press books may be ordered through booksellers or by contacting:

Balboa Press
A Division of Hay House
1663 Liberty Drive
Bloomington, IN 47403
www.balboapress.com
844-682-1282

Print information available on the last page.

ISBN: 978-1-9822-6546-5 (sc)
ISBN: 978-1-9822-6545-8 (hc)
ISBN: 978-1-9822-6547-2 (e)

Library of Congress Control Number: 2021907277

Balboa Press rev. date: 04/15/2021

CONTENTS

INTRODUCTION

I have always had a passion for healthy living. Even as a child, I remember thinking to myself that there must be a way to stay healthy and not get sick, even from colds. From early in my childhood, I said that I wanted to be a doctor because I wanted to help people feel better. I used to spend my summers in high school shadowing doctors at clinics, and I volunteered as a candy striper at a hospital for a few years. However, when I was sixteen, my family was in a terrible car accident, and that changed my entire perception of medicine and what helping people feel better really meant to me.

Everyone was fine, but my mom ended up with a severe nerve pinch in her shoulder. It was so bad that no one could even touch her without her being in excruciating pain. I saw my parents deal with the insurance bureaucracy to get her the right tests and treatment. Once she was diagnosed, doctors presented her with an option for surgery that had a very small chance of working. In fact, the odds of paralysis or her living with the pain were higher than the odds of the surgery actually making her better. While all this was going on, my mom was on painkillers, which had side effects, for which she then had more medication.

Then a family friend recommended yoga. Although the doctors advised against any physical activity, my parents thought, *What's the worst that could happen?* and decided to try it out. Within six weeks, she felt completely better. Medical doctors could not help her over a span of six months, but my yoga teacher helped her in six weeks. This was when I began wondering about the benefits of alternative health and whether there was another way to help people. My mom made a choice, and she chose to try something new to help herself feel better.

Thus began my journey into the world of alternative and complementary medicine. I found Maharishi University of Management, now known as Maharishi International University, which was the only accredited institution at the time that offered a bachelor's degree to study Ayurveda. Ayurveda is a form of complementary or natural approach to medicine that originated in India. In Sanskrit, Ayu means life and Veda means knowledge. Thus Ayurveda is the knowledge of life in particular to health and wellbeing. During my undergraduate years of study, I trained to become a classical hatha yoga teacher with the same teacher who helped my mom. After graduation, I continued to work in the fields of Ayurveda, health education, health promotion, and nutrition. I even went on to earn my master's degree in holistic health education with an emphasis in holistic nutrition.

I started integrating Ayurveda with modern science very early in my career. While I was studying for my bachelor's degree, I gave lectures at a local spa and wellness centre about Ayurveda's six tastes and how they influence digestion. Each of the doshas in Ayurveda and the six tastes have their specific functions that play a role when it comes to digestion. Being the lecturer allowed me to integrate and present the knowledge in a way to which the attendees could relate. After earning my bachelor's degree, the first Ayurvedic clinic I worked full-time at was in Encinitas, California. There, I began working mostly with clients who had neurological conditions, such as multiple sclerosis, and thus began my specialisation in autoimmune conditions using Ayurveda and modern science.

When I went on to study for my master's degree at John F. Kennedy University, all my professors were supportive and knew how important it was to me to integrate the knowledge of modern nutrition with Ayurveda. They helped me every step of the way. I have always loved learning about both Eastern and Western approaches to health. Blending the two has been a real passion, and I have seen first-hand the positive difference it makes for my clients.

Throughout my years as a clinical nutritionist, Ayurvedic health specialist, yoga teacher, and health educator, I have seen the consistent pattern that healthy results are due to the choices that are made. My clients achieve results, whether it is improved skin, healthier digestion, balanced blood sugar levels, or weight loss, because they choose to make the changes and commit to living healthier lifestyles. Life is full of choices. Waking up in the morning in itself is a choice. From there, your morning routine, what you choose to wear, whether you exercise, what food you eat—everything is a choice. Your health is about how you choose to live your life. When life throws you curveballs, again, you have a choice as to how you handle it. Everything that I am about to share with you in this book is about how the choices you make influence your health and well-being. As you realise the importance of the decisions you make that influence your health, this book will also help you make healthier choices in a way that is simple and practical.

This book is not about achieving perfectionism. We live in a world where everyone and everything needs to be presented perfectly. However, *perfect* has different meanings to different people. *Think Healthy, Choose Healthy* is about making healthy changes in a way that is doable. Being healthy is not about being able to do it all, but rather about how even the smallest of choices can make a big difference to how you feel. Even at times when you feel that you have no choice, you still do in some ways, which I will demonstrate. Healthy eating and living was never meant to be overwhelming or even stressful. I will show you how to be "healthy" in a more simplified way.

YOU STRUGGLE BECAUSE YOU ARE OUT OF BALANCE

The truth is you are here because you feel that something needs to change. Whatever it is that you are doing is not working for you anymore, and it's time to find a new approach. Perhaps you are under high amounts of stress or are completely lacking in energy. Perhaps your digestive system is not working, and food does not sit well with you. Perhaps you are constantly getting ill or are struggling to lose weight. Whatever it is, something simply is not right, and you want to feel healthier again. Being healthy is not about weight loss or even looking a certain way. Being healthy is about feeling good within yourself. This may range from sleeping better to having more fun, having a stronger metabolism, or simply having more energy. You want a new approach that is simple to adapt into your already busy lifestyle. I am here to offer you exactly that. Follow my approach, and you will soon realise that healthy living is actually quite simple.

More often than not, the struggle with health starts with something very subtle. For some, it starts with an occasional headache or achy back. For others, this could mean the odd heartburn, indigestion, or occasional constipation. These rare occurrences slowly begin to overtake your life. All of a sudden you cannot sleep no matter what you do. Perhaps you cannot eat a meal without going to the toilet straight afterwards. For some reason, you always feel thirsty. Or how about this one: you cannot wake up in the morning no matter how many hours of sleep you get. All these are real health challenges.

Notice how I did not mention weight. Yes, you should be at a healthy weight, but it is up to you and your doctor or health professional to decide what a healthy weight means to you. The body mass index, more commonly known as BMI, is a standard height-weight chart that is the same for men and women whether you are eighteen old or eighty years old. This chart does not account for age, ethnicity, health history, lifestyle, fitness, or diet. BMI also does not account for actual fat mass or muscle mass, and therefore it can be potentially misleading in terms of defining how healthy you actually are.[1] Weight is not the only factor that defines health. However, how you feel can define your health. For example, if you feel that you are overweight and would like to lose weight, then this is a real health concern that you need to address. I always tell my clients that unless there is a clinical reason to lose weight, weight loss in itself is a personal choice. In fact, there is an entire nutrition sector dedicated to the model of "health at every size". Also known as HAES, this model is one that accepts body diversity and teaches that people of all sizes and shapes are also healthy. They promote staying active and eating well within your means, but they also teach body acceptance and embracing who you are.[2] Your health is not solely defined by your BMI or appearance. There are a variety of considerations to make in addition to muscle and fat percentage. That includes but is not limited to inflammation levels, cholesterol, blood sugar, hormones, sleep, fitness, and of course nutrition levels.

Then there is the opposite of weight loss, which is weight gain. Some people want to put on weight, whether it's because they feel that they are too skinny, want to gain muscle mass, or have an underlying health condition. This book can definitely help with weight gain too. Or you may feel you are missing something in your life, but you may not be able to point to what the lack is. Something needs to change. You simply do not feel as healthy as you used to. As we go on this journey of making healthy living simpler and creating new habits, you will also have the chance to learn more about yourself. After all, it is your life and your health, so you must do what works best for you.

I truly believe that your food choices make a difference in how you feel. The classic saying goes, "You are what you eat." This is 100 per cent true, and your dietary choices are a direct reflection of that in some way, shape, or form. Your health can affect how you feel mentally, physically, emotionally, and even spiritually. Food to people is like petrol for a car: you must have it to be able to function. If you put the wrong type of fuel in the car, it can cause a lot of damage and cost a lot of money to fix. Likewise, if you put too much of unhealthy foods into your body, it will cost you a lot of time and money to correct it. Every person needs protein, carbohydrates, and fats to be able to function; they are fuel for your body. These are known as macronutrients and can be calculated to see exactly how much you need to meet your health goals. However, as my clients will tell you, counting your macronutrients is not a sustainable way to make healthy changes. Without counting, you still need all three for your body to have all essential nutrients directly from food.

Carbohydrates seem to have a bad reputation for no good reason. Not all carbohydrates are bad. When most people think of carbohydrates, or carbs, they think of breads, pasta, and baked pastries. However, there is a lot more to it than that. Carbs are also all your fruits, vegetables, and whole grains, which are foods that are essential to healthy living. Officially, there are two types of carbohydrates, simple and complex. Those are further divided into numerous categories. To keep it basic, simple carbs are sugars, whereas complex carbs are starches and fibre. The simple sugars can be further divided into two categories of natural and refined sugars. Natural sugars are those that come from fruit and dairy. Refined sugar is table sugar and other sweeteners such as honey, and it can be found in fruit juices, pastries, cakes, and biscuits. Starchy carbohydrates are items such as rice, pulses, and potatoes.

Fibre containing carbohydrates are whole grains, nuts, seeds, legumes, and vegetables. There is an overlap between starchy and fibrous carbohydrates, so foods can be in multiple categories.

In terms of functioning, carbohydrates contain essential nutrients, so you need to ensure that you eat from all the main categories. The consumption of carbohydrates directly affects your energy levels because carbs are the best source of energy. Simple or natural sugars are easy to digest and are almost instantly passed into your bloodstream. This is why fruits and dairy can also satisfy your sugar needs, but they do not necessarily provide a sustained amount of energy because they are quickly absorbed. However, natural sugars are needed to provide the body with energy, and they also contain either fibre or protein. The important thing to note here is that simple sugars are fine to have as long as you consume them in moderation.

Your refined or processed carbohydrates are still considered to be simple sugars, but they contain little to no nutritional value; often they are high in calories and contain little to no fibre. Studies show that a diet high in refined sugars can lead to numerous health conditions such as type 2 diabetes, weight gain, obesity, high cholesterol, digestive issues, trouble with sleep, and nutrient deficiencies. Refined sugar consumption should be kept to an absolute minimum.

Complex carbohydrates should become your best friend. These have a very rich nutritional value, and as complex carbs, they are rich in fibre; they take longer to digest and therefore keep you fuller for longer. They are a more sustained source of energy and satiety. The key factor here is that the more complex carbs you eat, the less likely you are to crave simple or refined carbohydrates.

Next up is protein, which is an essential nutrient. Protein is made up of amino acids, which are known as the building blocks. There are over twenty different amino acids, but only nine are essential. This means that you need to consume the following nine amino acids through your food: histidine, isoleucine, leucine, lysine, methionine, phenylalanine, threonine, tryptophan, and valine.[3] Your body can make the rest of the amino acid types, so you do not need to have those through food or supplementation. There is a difference between meat and dairy sources of protein and vegetarian sources of protein. Fish, poultry, meat, eggs, and dairy are considered to be complete protein sources. This means that each individual product contains all nine essential amino acids. However, protein sources such as beans, legumes, nuts, seeds, and whole grains are incomplete protein sources. This means that you must combine any two together to make it a complete protein source. If you only have one, then that means you will not get all your essential amino acids. Vegetarians and especially vegans need to be extra cautious about this. For example, if you have a lentil for dinner, be sure to couple it with brown rice so that you are getting all your essential amino acids. Protein can also be used by the body to be utilised as energy, however it is inefficient. It takes the body four times more effort to turn protein into energy compared to carbohydrates. Therefore high-protein meals or shakes should be avoided before exercise.

Protein is excellent to consume after any form of exercise because it helps with muscle building and tissue repair. However, too little or too much protein can have adverse effects. For example, too little protein can cause weakness in muscles as well as negatively impact the health of your hair, nails, and skin. Aside from causing weakened bones, a protein deficiency may weaken your immune system, which would make you more susceptible to developing infections.[4] Too much protein can impair kidney functioning and may cause kidney stones. High consumption of meat, especially red meat, can cause high cholesterol and is also known to increase risk of colon cancer.[5]

Fats also have a bad reputation, but they really are not that bad. Having too much or too little fat can affect energy levels and nutrient absorption. Fats are a must as part of a balanced diet. They provide insulation to the body and structure to all the cell membranes. They transport all fat-soluble vitamins such as vitamins A, D, E, and K. This means that without fat, your body cannot absorb these nutrients. Fats can be categorised into three main categories: saturated fats, unsaturated fats, and trans fats. Saturated fats are actually a healthy source of cholesterol, and you need some saturated fat because cholesterol is what makes your sex and stress hormones. Some sources of saturated fats are meat, poultry, eggs, dairy, and coconut oil. Unsaturated fats are your omega 3s, 6s, and 9s. These are essential fats that must be obtained through food, meaning your body cannot make these. They protect the heart, are considered to be anti-inflammatory, and are excellent for arthritis, heart disease, diabetes, and autoimmune conditions. Some sources include salmon, halibut, sardines, flaxseeds, chia seeds, olives, nut oils, and avocados. You must consume both saturated and unsaturated fats, however it should be in moderation.

The type of fats that you want to avoid are the trans fats, which are essentially damaged or bad fats. These are the ones that have been artificially made by the food industry. They create free radicals, cause oxidative damage, and increase inflammation within the body. The liver has a tough time processing them. Although they are often made from vegetable sources, they are designed to mimic saturated fats and have a longer shelf life. Hydrogenated oils are an example of trans fats. Worst of all, trans fats prevent the absorption of nutrients.

I just introduced a lot of basic information about carbohydrates, proteins, and fats. The reason for this is that I want to emphasise the importance of having all three in your daily life, but of course in moderation. Having too much or too little of any macronutrient can cause more damage than good. For example, I had a client diagnosed with irritable bowel syndrome; let's call her Laurie. Her main problem was severe constipation and heartburn. After doing some reading online and taking the advice of her friends, she decided to become vegan and eliminate a variety of foods, including gluten, dairy, soy, nuts, spicy foods, and nightshades. Laurie eliminated all these foods for several weeks, but not only did her symptoms not get any better, they actually got worse, and she started to put on weight. That was when she was introduced to me. It turned out she was eating too many packaged and processed foods with lots of additives in order to stay away from the foods she eliminated, and she was missing her essential amino acids and other key nutrients. Laurie and her friends meant well, but in the end she did not need to eliminate any of the foods at all. All she needed to do was repair her digestive system, which we did, and now she eats everything in moderation and knows exactly how to keep her digestion strong.

In addition to your diet, your lifestyle or daily routine can also lead you to being off balance. Your choices outside of food also make a huge difference and these areas are often neglected. Yes, food is of the utmost importance, but so is sleep and how you spend your time. We all have an internal body clock within us, known as circadian rhythm. It plays a crucial role that helps regulate the sleep and wake cycles along with hormones, eating habits, digestion, body temperature, and other bodily functions.[6] Scientists know for a fact that circadian rhythms influence and determine sleep patterns. The hormone that induces sleep, melatonin, begins to release when there is less light. However, with indoor lights and heavy screen time, this can delay the release of melatonin, which can be one of the causes of insomnia; it may cause you to not feel sleep near bedtime.

Sleep is very important, and people know how awful they feel when they do not get enough of it. Lack of sleep results in low energy levels, weakened immunity, trouble concentrating, and increased mood swings. It is important to identify how much sleep you need and then ensure you are able to get plenty of it. When sleep routine is disturbed, the circadian rhythms are disturbed, and as mentioned earlier, circadian rhythms are responsible for much more than just your sleep. A missed night of sleep here or there will not cause much damage except for the fact that you may just feel overly tired and cannot focus. However, chronic sleep deprivation can cause more serious health challenges such as obesity, heart disease, diabetes, and high blood pressure. Even too much sleep can result in feeling lethargic or having a slow metabolism.

Circadian rhythm, your internal body clock, also thrives on routine and having consistent sleep and wake habits.

An imbalanced diet and insufficient sleep can make you already feel on edge. Adding high stress levels to the mix can really make you feel that you are out of control with your own health. Stress is something that everyone experiences, but it is about how you manage it. When your stress levels rise and leave you feeling out of control, you may have physical, mental, or emotional symptoms. Physical symptoms of high stress may include headaches, muscle pain or tension, stomach problems, chest pain, and racing heartbeat. Mental and emotional symptoms include irritability, trouble sleeping, difficulty concentrating, feeling overwhelmed, overly worried, forgetfulness, overeating, skipping meals, anxiety, and even depending on alcohol or drugs, to name a few. Ultimately, stress can really affect how you feel, and you will notice the symptoms manifest in a variety of ways.

Stress response involves the nervous system, particularly the peripheral nervous system. This further divides into two more categories: the somatic nervous system, which controls the voluntary movement, and the autonomic nervous system, which controls the involuntary movement. Let's focus on the autonomic nervous system, which is what regulates many of the automatic functions of the body such as the heart beating, respiration, and digestive system. This can be divided further into another two categories, the sympathetic and parasympathetic nervous system. The sympathetic nervous system is known as the "fight or flight" mode, which activates when the body is under any form of stress. The parasympathetic nervous system is known as the "rest or digest" mode because that is what keeps the body calm and preserves energy.[7]

It is important to know this because in a way, at any given moment, your body is either "resting or digesting" or is in "fight or flight" mode. You cannot have both active at the same time. Therefore when many people are under stress, they may feel that they cannot relax, or their digestive system feels off balance. When under any type of stress, your body will use as much energy as it can and will place all the attention on resolving that stress. This means that if you are constantly under stress, the rest of the body will suffer because the other organs will not receive the full attention that they deserve. A client of mine, Paul, suffered from gastrointestinal problems for many years and was also gaining weight. He worked as an accountant in a large firm. With a thorough health history and understanding his diet and lifestyle, I came to the conclusion that it was in fact that his job that was making his digestion worse. He could not leave his job, but he learned to manage his stress through nutrition and meditation, which helped him feel better and lose weight without even having to try.

More often than not, high stress also leads to a feeling of excess fatigue. The nervous system will do its best to balance the stress, but if you allow the stress to continue, then other areas of your body will suffer such as your mental health or your digestive system. In particular, one area that is getting more attention these days is the health of your adrenal glands. Excessive and high amounts of stress can lead to adrenal insufficiency. Your two small adrenal glands sit on top of the kidneys and produce many hormones including cortisol and adrenaline. Cortisol is released every time you feel stress. The theory is that there is only so much cortisol your body can release before your adrenal glands feel depleted from constantly releasing hormones to help you regain a balanced state of health. Adrenal insufficiency is known to cause low energy, depression, mood swings, brain fog, and other symptoms that are also related to high stress levels. The main point is that stress in general upsets the homeostasis, or balance, within your body on all levels of mental, physical, and spiritual well-being

Take a moment to engage in a self-reflection exercise and answer the following questions regarding how you react to stress and anxiety. I highly recommend that you write your answers on a sheet of paper, but you are of course welcome to use a phone, tablet, or computer.

- How do you react to stress and anxiety?
- How do you clear your mind?
- How do you stay positive?
- Is the glass half-full or half-empty?
- Is there a problem?
- Do you feel that you have enough time in the day to get everything done?

Do not worry if you do not have the answers to all the questions, or even if you are unsure how to answer them. Answer them the best you can, and you can refer to these questions later.

Ayurveda has the perfect answer to why you may struggle with your health or suffer from any disease. For those who have never come across Ayurveda, this is a form of medicine that originated in India, and it is considered to be one of the original forms of medicine in the East. Ayurveda is becoming increasingly popular, especially in the Western world, because it has much to offer. *Ayu* in Sanskrit means life, and *veda* means knowledge. Together, Ayurveda is considered to be the total knowledge of life, especially in terms of your health. Ayurveda believes that "overuse, underuse, and misuse, of time, senses, and action" are what lead to disease and imbalances.[8]

Moderation is the key to healthy living, but when something is done too much or too little, that is where imbalance rises. For example, staying up late to binge-watch a television show is both an overuse and misuse of your time, senses, and action. The time you should be sleeping is now being used to watch a show that is over stimulating your senses. The action is that you choose to stay up late because you really want to see what happens next in the show. Staying up late and not getting enough sleep can weaken your immune system. Another example is skipping meals because you are too busy working. By skipping a meal, you are misusing and underusing your time, senses, and action. Senses would relate to your sense of taste because you are depriving yourself of food and essential nutrients so you can work. Not enough food can also cause stress within your body and upset your digestive, nervous, and immune systems.

You cannot separate just time, senses, or actions. At least two of the three are connected at any given point. Similarly, underuse, misuse, and overuse are all connected as well. Every choice you make will either work in your favour or work against you. How you choose to spend your time and what you do with your time will make a difference in terms of how you feel. This is where you also want to begin to think about how you use all five of your senses within all the tasks that you do every day. Even looking at a computer screen for too long or reading a book without taking any breaks is overuse and misuse of your time, senses, and action. Your eyes and brain need a break, and we have all heard about how sitting for too long can cause back pain or increase your weight. Spending too much time planning, problem-solving, daydreaming, thinking in general, entertaining random thoughts, working, or worrying is also a overuse, underuse, and misuse of time, senses, and action. All your actions have either positive or negative consequences, so it really does come back to what is best for you as an individual. Your health is about finding the right balance and is a result of the choices you make.

GET TO KNOW YOURSELF AND LEARN MORE ABOUT YOU

Before you can make any dietary or lifestyle changes, you must learn about yourself. Changes work best if you start from your place of comfort, knowledge, and acceptance. This means that not all changes will happen overnight, but in order to make changes, you must know and recognise both your strengths and weaknesses. Therefore, take a few moments and answer the following questions.

- Thinking of your busiest day, what is your routine?
- What do you do for you?
- What are some of your hobbies and interests?
- Imagine your ideal day. What would you do?

The truth of the matter is that no matter where you are in terms of your health and overall well-being, you must prioritise self-care. This should be one of those things that is nonnegotiable, like brushing your teeth. Self-care is a basic necessity and looks different for everybody. Self-care is also one of the hardest to incorporate, but it is the most important. It's easy to neglect because it only involves yourself, and more often than not, it may feel like a selfish act. However, it is not a selfish act because the act of self-care is what allows you to care for others. As the classic saying goes, you cannot give from an empty cup." Let's say that you left in a rush because you are feeling stressed. You are out and about with your child, who asks you for some water. You open your bag to find that the water bottle is empty because you forgot to fill it up, and what's worse, you left your wallet at home. Now, there is no water for you or your child until you get back home. The point is that if you do not take the time to fill up your water bottle, you will not be able to help others if you do not keep your own resources full.

One of the factors that make self-care easier is acceptance. Once you accept that self-care is essential, then you will begin to think more about it. You also need it the most when you feel exhausted or overwhelmed. Therefore, when you feel like there is too much to do and not enough time, accept that this is the case. Accept that life is challenging at the moment. When life gets difficult, it's best to look forward and not back. Things are not the same, so don't force yourself to keep them the same. In order to prioritise self-care, create a new plan and reprioritise. And in order to reprioritise, create new boundaries. Carve out some time for yourself and remember you must help yourself first before helping others.

This all sounds easy, but in order to put it into practice, you must learn about what works for you and what does not. Think about your feelings and answer the following questions. Write it down on the same sheet as before as this is also a journaling exercise.

What activity do you do, and what do you eat, when you are feeling the following things?

-   bored
-   happy
-   angry
-   lonely
-   tired
-   depressed

- celebratory
- hungry
- sad

Knowing how you respond to various emotions and feelings is a great place to start. For example, when you are feeling lonely, you may sit and cry. In an act of self-care, when you feel lonely, it may be a good idea to start thinking about other activities you could do instead that will help nourish yourself, like calling a friend or going for a walk. Other factors that you want to make note of is what makes you happy and what makes you sad. Create a list and write it out. In the process, engage all five of your senses. For example, for the sense of taste, think about your favourite foods. Then list at least five items that you would love to eat anytime, anywhere. Repeat this for the senses of smell, touch, sight, and sound. Smell could be any fragrance, touch could be your favourite material of clothing to wear, sight is something you love to look at for hours at a time, and sound is your favourite sound of nature or music. This is an endless activity, but take the time to make a list. You do not have to limit yourself to five things, but it's a good starting point. Take a few moments to engage your senses and write down what you are feeling.

Once you learn about how your senses are best engaged, then you should also learn about your favourite drinks, people, places, books, and anything else that you can think of. All these factors play a role in your health and well-being. Anything that makes you happy will help promote good health, whereas factors that cause you stress will weaken your health.

Another great technique to apply to learn more about yourself is to use mindfulness. Mindfulness is a very hot-button word at the moment and gets used by a variety of professionals. Mindfulness is the act of being intensely aware of what you are sensing and feeling at every moment without any interpretation of judgement. It is the act of allowing you to just be and experience stillness. The classic example often seen is when you are walking your dog. Are you simply observing nature around you, are you thinking about the one hundred other things you need to do with a constant stream of thoughts running through your mind, so much so that you do not even notice the beauty of nature around you?

Mindfulness is also about paying attention to yourself and to your environment. It is looking and reflecting inside while looking at the world straight on. It is about being interested and curious to learn more about yourself. The more you pay attention to your mind and to your body, the more you will learn about yourself. Ultimately, it is about living in the present moment. The past is gone and the future is uncertain, but what you do have right now is the moment. Never be afraid to ask and check in with yourself to see how you are feeling in this very moment. By engaging in this mindful behaviour, you will soon become more aware of your thoughts, words, and actions.

As you learn more about yourself you will realise that you are in the driver's seat. Nobody else is responsible for your health, and your health is literally in your hands. Yes, others can influence you, but for the most part you can choose your company. Every day you make decisions, from what time you wake up to what you wear, where you go, and what you eat. Your life is a culmination of all the choices that you have made. Many of the choices that you make are automatic. You may not even see them as a choice that makes a difference. For example, you may choose tea over coffee or coffee over tea, but to you, it does not matter, and there may be no long-term repercussions. Nevertheless, it is still a choice. At that point, you begin to think, "Should I have chosen to drink water instead of the tea or coffee?" Your health is a result of the choices that you have made.

With your choices being central to your overall well-being, take the time to invest in yourself. This relates back to self-care. Expand your horizons and continue to learn. Explore hobbies and other areas that may be of interest to you. Take official or even unofficial courses. Get the degree that you always wanted. Learn more about a subject simply because you want to, not because you have to. This is the purpose of learning more about yourself. It is an opportunity to explore more of what makes you happy and engage in an activity that brings you joy. This is where you also learn about what is important to you and where your priorities lie.

A good chunk of living a healthy lifestyle is also about creating healthy boundaries. In order to do so, you must know where your comforts lie, what are you willing to explore, and where you absolutely do not want to go to. Therefore, you have to take personal responsibility—nobody can do this for you. For example, if you have a casein allergy, which means you are allergic to dairy, then you know that for you to stay healthy, you must say no to dairy at any cost. This is your boundary. However, let's say you have a mild digestive intolerance to gluten; then you may think to yourself, "Sometimes I can have it and sometimes not." In any given situation, you decide whether or not it is worth having gluten.

Other ways to create healthy boundaries is to ask for help. People often perceive asking for help as sign of weakness, but that is actually not true. Asking for help is a sign of strength because it shows that you are aware of what you can do on your own and what you need some assistance with. In fact, asking for help and getting others you trust involved can even help you get things done faster. There is nothing wrong with asking for help. Likewise, it is just as important to be able to say no. As much as you want to please people and make others happy, sometimes you simply have to say no. Saying no does not mean that you are unwilling to help; it means that at the moment you do not have the capacity to be able to help. How many times have you agreed to help someone, and all the while you are feeling overly stretched for time and have put yourself out of your way? We have all been there. The theory here is that no one should overstretch oneself to help others.

This does not mean that you constantly ask help from others without returning the favour. It simply means that you treat others the way you would like to be treated. Ask for help and help others, but sometimes it is perfectly acceptable to say no without giving an explanation. When I first started my business, I used to say yes to every opportunity that came my way, whether it was paid or free. Then I was overly stretched and completely lost my focus. That was when I realised I needed to say no at times and keep my priorities clear.

As you create healthy boundaries, this also means choosing to leave work at a certain time and, once you are home, switching off from work. If you work from home, it may mean having a dedicated workspace, and once you leave that workspace, work is left there. From an efficiency perspective, taking breaks and working smartly is more effective. Studies show that working longer hours makes you slower at the work you do and therefore makes you less productive. Although initially you start off being productive, after you reach your threshold of about forty to fifty hours for the week, productivity begins to decline. The more overtime you do, you may as well not work. That is how unproductive you become.[9] Therefore, it is important to have working or professional boundaries as well as personal boundaries. Know what you can handle and what you cannot. When it is too much for you, speak up and stand up for yourself. Others cannot know what your limits are unless you tell them. Ensure to communicate your needs. If there is too much work on your plate, then ask for help. If you feel that you are taking home too much work which does not leave you with enough time to do what you want to in your personal life, you must share that. Expressing your needs is a big step in creating healthy boundaries.

As you begin to think about self-care and creating those healthy boundaries, be sure to manage your time. The truth is you have the time for anything that is important to you. Have you noticed that sports fans always have time to watch the games, and some people always have time to exercise, cook, or read? Ultimately, people always have time for something that is important to them.

Grab your piece of paper and note down what is of importance to you. What do you enjoy? What do you like to do? If you had an extra hour in a day, how would you spend it? These are very important questions to ask yourself as you reprioritise and make time for yourself. Everything outlined thus far and later in this book will come back to time, priorities, and choices. What do you have time for?

I would like you to reflect and think about how you spend your time. Keep track of your working and nonworking hours. What do you really do all day? Do this activity for a few days, and you will see the gaps in your day, or places where you could have improved productivity. It may also be possible that you do not have any gaps during the day. This is where you need to take a step back and reassess your priorities. Is your busy-ness really worth it? It is also important to take breaks regardless of how busy you are. Working constantly slows down productivity, so take the time to recharge and reset. This is where self-care can slide in.

Your time is valuable to you, and you get to choose how you spend it. When learning about a new routine or incorporating new ways of self-care, it is helpful to work with a schedule. Create a schedule; whether it is on a device or in a calendar, write down your daily routine. Then stick to it. Be flexible with your routine but stay firm to your priorities. For example, if you have scheduled yourself in for a massage, but then a client wants to meet with you at the same time, do not reschedule your massage. Simply ask the client to meet you at another time. More often than not, the client will be more than willing to accommodate your schedule. At the same time, keep in mind you do not owe anyone an explanation of what you are doing with your time. Your self-care time is precious, and you do not have to share with everyone what you do.

I have a yoga student who is a director at a major company, and she has to work long hours. She has been coming to my classes for years, and after one of my daily yoga challenges, she practices nearly every day. However, her yoga practice is very personal for her. On the busiest days in the office, she closes the blinds in her office, locks the door, and does her personal yoga practice for half an hour. Her personal assistant knows what she does, but she does not tell anyone else because that time is nonnegotiable. If others found out, she does not want the pressure of anyone knowing that she does yoga; more specifically, she does not want others to think that this is "just yoga", which she can do later. For her, this is not "just yoga" because her mind and body need this to keep up with the demands of her job. Likewise, I would like you to think of what form of self-care is so important to you that it is nonnegotiable. Consider ways you can incorporate it into your daily routine.

If you currently do not have any hobbies or feel that time is a real issue, create a bucket list of hobby ideas that you would like to try if you had no constraints whatsoever. This means in an ideal world, if you had the infinite time and resources, how would you like to spend it? What activity would bring you joy? If time is an issue, think about times in the day when you can get away for a few moments. For example, I have clients who do stretches while waiting for the kettle to boil, and some spend a few extra minutes in the bathroom every day to do some reading. Be honest about what activities would bring a smile to your face and would also take care of you at the same time, and where you can, make the time.

DIETS DON'T WORK

None of my clients diet. I have been practicing nutrition and Ayurveda for many years, and I have never had a single one of my clients diet to lose weight. Sure, I have had clients asking to be put on a calorie-controlled diet or to try a particular diet, but usually by the end of the first session, I have talked them out of it and fully convinced them that diets do not work, but nutrition does work. Everybody is different, and what works for one person may not work for another person. Similarly, some people get instant results, whereas for others it takes time.

This is why I love Ayurveda so much. Ayurveda has always taken into account that each person is different and that there is no such thing as a one-size-fits-all model. Each person has his or her own unique body type. In fact, there is now an official branch of medicine, known as functional medicine, that teaches doctors to treat each patient individually and not the same as the hundreds of others they see with the same disease. Functional medicine has another division, which is functional nutrition. This is one of the branches I studied when I did my master's degree. Functional nutrition recognises that each individual will have different nutritional needs and will need to find his or her own balance in different ways, which may include the need to heal the digestive system. Functional nutrition goes beyond looking at nutritional deficiencies. Rather, it works with nutrients in a way

21

of synergy by taking into account a variety of other factors such as genetics, lifestyle, and environment.[10] One could say that functional nutrition is a holistic approach to the entire field of dietetics.

When it comes to achieving any health goal, there are a multitude of factors that need incredible consideration. Some of these factors are digestion, hydration, exercise, level of activity, health history, mental health, physical health, emotional health, health goals, dietary intake, iron levels, inflammation levels, and nutritional deficiencies. Think of it this way: if we take two people who have type 2 diabetes, and both are 5'8" and weigh 78 kilogrammes, they cannot be treated in the exact same way. In both cases, their medical histories are different, as are their daily lifestyle, jobs, income, families, and support systems. Everything is different, so how can the same type 2 diabetes diet work for them?

Nutritional deficiencies must be considered when changing any dietary plan. How many fad diets out there actually take into account the micronutrients? Vitamins and minerals are micronutrients, and they must be consumed through diet or supplementation because your body cannot make them. I have also heard people say, "It is OK; I take a multivitamin every day," and in their eyes, this makes up for their unhealthy dietary choices. However, a multivitamin is only as good as one's daily diet. Multivitamins and other health supplements are good as a top-up, but they are not an alternative. I often cringe when my fitness clients take large amounts of protein shakes because their personal trainer told them to. Many mainstream shakes they drink are often loaded with added sugars or sweeteners along with nonessential amino acids, which burden the body more. Too much protein is not good for you either.

Another reason why diets do not work is that dietary beliefs and any food allergies or intolerances need to be accounted for. For example, being vegetarian or vegan and having any sort of underlying allergy needs to be addressed. If you are allergic to chicken—and I have clients who are—then any diet that promotes eating meat would not be suitable for you. Rather than going on a diet, it is more important to learn about which foods work well for you and which do not.

Ultimately, diets do not provide long-term results. Most of the time, diets do provide instant short-term results, but remember that Rome was not built in a day. Whether it's weight loss or improving your digestion, think about how long the problem has been around for. If you have been struggling with your health for years, you cannot fix the problem overnight. Rather, it will take time, and you need to be patient with yourself. The trouble with diets is that they are very short-term focused with no information on how to proceed or continue long-term. Eventually you will return to your former dietary and lifestyle habits, and then you will go back to how you were feeling before. Therefore with weight loss, once you go on a fad diet, you are likely to put the weight back—plus more—once you come off of the diet.[11] Keep in mind the faster you lose the weight, the more challenging it is to maintain that new weight, and thus you are more likely to gain back the weight.

Diets are too restrictive. The truth is you can only do intermittent fasting for so long before you begin to feel tired and calorie deficient, which will ultimately lead to nutritional deficiencies. When you are too restrictive with what you consume, regardless of specific type of diet, this can lead to food cravings, weakened digestion and metabolism, low energy, or mood swings. With that said, not all diets are terrible. Some have their merits, such as the ones that have their foundation in Ayurveda, or the Schwarzbein Principle, which helps regulate blood sugar levels, or the metabolic typing diet, which also takes into account individual body types. None of these diets are restrictive but rather aim to find a good balance of macronutrients and micronutrients to restore health in the bigger picture.

When choose or selecting a dietary plan, you must consider the amount of flexibility it has to offer. Diets can be difficult to maintain because choices are not always available. Many people also face the challenge of what to eat when eating out or going out for social events and gatherings. Take for example the FODMAP diet, which is a specialty diet for those suffering from severe irritable bowel syndrome. Although it is very helpful, it can be potentially very restrictive. However, it is a good one to follow temporarily until you figure which foods are causing you trouble. Then as you slowly introduce foods back in, you will then have more options. But diets such as those should only be done under the guidance of a health professional because when done on one's own, they can be even more restrictive than what they need to be.

To be honest, the only thing worse than dieting itself is calorie counting. Even when you are not aiming to lose weight, calorie counting is not an exact science. Not only is it time-consuming, but it doesn't always work. Weighing foods and measuring all the time is also not sustainable. Although there are suggested portion sizes, meal sizes vary from person to person. Furthermore, in an attempt to eat fewer calories, you often end up eating more artificial and processed foods. In order to make them taste better, low-calorie foods are often laced with artificial additives and processed foods.

When selecting foods, it is important to know more than just the number of calories. What you really need to know is its nutritional value. How much goodness is in there in terms of vitamins and minerals? Is it as close to natural form as you can get? You also want to know the fibre content along with any added sugars or other ingredients. The best way to keep it simple is to eat as cleanly as possible and look at the quality of the ingredients, not just the quantity. For example, let's take a can of Coke. A 330 mL can of original coke has 139 calories and no nutritional value whatsoever. For the same number of calories, you could have 33 grammes of dried apricots with 33 grammes of almonds. Together, these contain fibre and protein, as well as naturally occurring sugar.

Here is an example of two diets that are about 1,600 calories a day.

Scenario A

1. Breakfast is a bowl of crunchy nut cornflakes with whole milk and a cup of coffee with milk and 1 sugar (300 calories)
2. Lunch is a ham, cheese, and pickle sandwich with a side of salted crisps (600 calories)
3. Afternoon snack is Belvita biscuits and a cup of coffee with milk and 1 sugar (200 calories)
4. Dinner is spaghetti bolognaise with beef (500 calories)

Scenario B

1. Breakfast is overnight oats with shredded coconut, raisins, nuts, and seeds made with almond milk, along with a cup of coffee with oat milk (400 calories)
2. Morning snack is an apple with almond butter (200 calories)
3. Lunch is a Greek chicken salad (350 calories)
4. Afternoon snack is Greek yogurt with berries, along with a cup of coffee containing oat milk (200 calories)
5. Dinner is chicken fajitas with pico de gallo and guacamole (450 calories)

Which one is healthier? Which one would be more nutritious?

This is what one of my clients used to eat (Scenario A) and what he now eats (Scenario B). Although both sets of daily food journals are about 1,600 calories, nutritionally they are polar opposites. Scenario A has very little fibre, has hardly any fruit or vegetables, and is high in sugar. In Scenario B, there are plenty of fruits, vegetables, whole grains, nuts, seeds, and protein, and overall it is a very healthy diet that is nutritionally rich. From the look of it, you can see that my client is now eating more often and feeling better for it as well. He is able to have two snacks a day rather than one, and there is plenty of variety within his diet. This is why not all calories are equal. Ultimately, what matters the most is the nutritional value of the food that you consume.

When shopping for food, I tell my clients to ignore the traffic light symbols in the front of the package, and for the majority, I also say look at the nutrition label as a secondary. What you really want to look at is the ingredients label. The ingredients is where you get the full story, and that is how you also know where your nutrients come from. Here is the actual information about what is inside the product you are about to eat. It's all good to know the number of calories and the grammes of carbohydrates, proteins, and fats, but what you really want to know is how much of the food is real. Ingredients are written in the order from the most to the least. For example, if you picked up a protein bar and the first ingredient is oats, then that means that there are more oats than anything else in the bar.

When reading ingredient labels, there are few key factors to consider. First is the length of the list of ingredients. Does your fruit-flavoured yogurt really need a list as long as your palm? What is in the ingredients? Do you recognise every single item listed? If you had the recipe, could you find all the ingredients in a common supermarket? How many chemicals or additives are in there? Just because a product looks healthy, that does not mean it is healthy. Food manufacturers are marketing their products to you when they design the front image. When reading the ingredients label, if sugar or a form of sugar or sweetener is one of the first three ingredients on the list, then it counts as a dessert. Ingredients that are labelled as an E number is also something to be cautious about. Not all E numbers are bad, but my theory is that if it's a real ingredient, why hide it behind a number? In fact, I love brands that often go out of their way to explain what a particular ingredient is and why it is even necessary to add it in. However, the lengthier the list of additives and preservatives, the more processed the food item is.

There is a movement on how being vegan is better for the environment. Yes, being vegan has its benefits, but the products you choose to eat also make a difference. Just because a product is labelled as being vegan does not make it healthier. Many vegan products are filled with so many different ingredients that it is highly processed. This is another instance when you want to consider whether or not the product is actually healthier. Low-fat, zero-calorie, and low-sugar foods may appear to be healthier, but the majority of the time, these foods are also laced with additives and are highly processed. Science does not guarantee that any of these foods are actually a healthier option. Many artificial sweeteners and additives are also quite controversial, and long-term safety is unknown. Functional nutrition knows that clean eating, or eating as close to natural and wholesome foods, is the healthier option. This means the less processed it is, the better the food is for you. Logically, this makes sense.

Nutritionists like me often believe that when people consume low-calorie or low-fat foods, they actually end up eating more but overall less nutritious foods. Sometimes a low-calorie option is simply not filling enough, where as you can easily substitute the hundred-calorie snack bar for an apple instead, thereby making it a healthier and more nutritious option. The other problem with having low-fat foods is that these foods are often fortified with added nutrients as well as other additives to make them tastier. Nutrients are much more absorbable when they are in their natural state as opposed to a synthetic form.

When it comes to food, healthy eating works regardless of health goals. In addition to eating well, the lifestyle needs to match up. It is nearly impossible to be 100 per cent healthy 100 per cent of the time. Due to the world we live in, unless you are living off grid and growing all your food in a purely sustainable way, this is not possible. Sure, you can come close to living like that, but it is quite challenging. Therefore the best way to live a healthier life is to follow the eighty-twenty (80/20) rule. This is the basic rule I have all my clients follow regardless of their health goals. This is also why my clients do not need to follow any particular diet for weight loss. This is my secret to success. The 80/20 rule is about eating healthy and sticking to your plan 80 per cent of the time; for the other 20 per cent of the time, you are free to deviate from the plan without feeling any sense of guilt. This rule means that you do not have to be too strict or hard on yourself. This is the rule that allows for flexibility and for you to enjoy the finer things in life. Eating only organic or following a strict regimen can make you feel your best while you are doing it, but as soon as you go off plan, it will affect your digestion and immunity. Being too strict can also cause a great deal of stress and anxiety because of the added layer of pressure to meet a certain criteria at all times. You must find the right balance. A balanced plan will have some wiggle room to help you cope with establishing the new habits.

I had a classmate during a course I took one summer who ate only organic and healthy foods. She followed a strict regimen of eating well, managing her stress, having a strict bed time, meditating daily without fail, and so forth. One could say that she had the best ideal daily routine in place for optimal health. However, when she would eat out or have a night of staying up even an hour past her bedtime, she would get extremely tired and sometimes fall ill. Ranging from constipation to actually getting the flu, her body was not ready to handle a curveball. This was because she did not allow for any flexibility.

The world we live in is filled with germs and chemicals within our environment and often in the food that is available. Therefore, even if it is a slight exposure, we all need to introduce our bodies to it. Some exposure will help keep our immune and digestive systems strong. Your body needs to be able to adapt and digest whatever you eat, and therefore as a bonus, your immune system will also be exposed to the chemicals and will know how to handle it. This is why it is important to follow the eighty-twenty rule. You need to allow for some flexibility within the choices that you make.

For example, children need to learn from early on about how to make healthy food choices within their school and home environment. They should be educated on knowing the difference between naturally occurring fructose in fruit and added sugar in biscuits. At some point in their lives, children will be exposed to unhealthy foods, so small exposure from early on will teach them how to make healthier choices.

Their bodies need to learn how to process and deal with such items from time to time. It is important to encourage children to select healthier foods and ensure they understand why. Teaching them about ingredients and quality of food will empower them.

When it comes to choosing healthy foods, I like to refer to Varsha's Healthy Scale. As I mentioned above, being super healthy all the time is not always practical. Sometimes the reality is that you may not even have the option for a fully healthy choice. This is where my scale comes in handy. Varsha's Healthy Scale is a one-to-five scale. One is a poor choice that is extremely unhealthy, whereas five is the healthiest option and is likely organic. When you are confronted with options as to what to eat or buy, use this scale and know that it is OK to choose a three or four; not all choices have to be a five. For example, let's say that you are out for dinner, and you had no say as to the location. You are at an Italian restaurant that only serves pizza and pasta. There is no real healthy options that you are fully satisfied about, however you end up picking the pasta with the most amount of vegetables, and you do not have any starters. The point is you still made the healthier choice out of the options you had—even though it was not the best choice, it was still a good choice. Fill your life with good and best options, not just best. At the same time, on the odd occasion, it is perfectly acceptable to have a one or two on the scale in the mix as well. Do not deprive yourself because that will create an unhealthy association with food.

Let's also leave the feeling of guilt behind if you eat something off plan. If you are going to eat something regardless of whether it is healthy for you, at the very least enjoy it rather than feeling guilty about it. Then accept that this is a choice that you made. If you feel that you are struggling because you indulge too much, then here is a list of questions to ask yourself before you make your decision to see whether or not it is worth eating that particular item.

1. Are you really hungry, or are you thirsty?
2. Are you bored?

3. Are there any emotions fuelling your hunger?
4. When did you last eat?
5. Are you sure you want to eat this?

Self-reflection and having that awareness are key to making healthier choices. If you go through all five of these questions before eating, especially if you find yourself snacking or nibbling on food too often, then this will help reframe your mindset and make you more aware of what is actually fuelling your food choices.

HOLISTIC APPROACH THAT ADDRESSES MIND, BODY, AND SPIRIT

The truth is that the mind, body, and spirit are intimately connected. In many ways, your mind makes the choices for your body, which reflects how you feel within yourself, which is known as the spirit. Your dietary and lifestyle choices strongly influence your overall state of being and how you feel at any given point. Spirit does not have to relate to religious or spiritual beliefs; rather, it is more of who you are at your core. This is why it is so important to learn more about yourself so that you can identify your strengths and weaknesses to improve your well-being.

The mind is most often associated with the brain and is known as the place that holds your thoughts; this is where all the thinking and processing happens. However, it is much more than that. The mind and your mental health are integral to your overall well-being. The mind has many qualities and attributes. This is where Ayurveda provides an excellent description of how the mind works through the concept of the three gunas. *Guna* is the Sanskrit word for quality. The three gunas are found within the mind, but they also found in the external environment. The three gunas are known as sattva, rajas, and tamas. Think of the three gunas as a traffic light. Sattva is known as purity and is the green light, signalling it is safe to move forward. Rajas means one should slow down and get ready to act or change direction, and it is the amber light. Tamas is the "stop and reassess" action, which is the red light. Just like you need the traffic lights to control the flow of cars, you also need the similar concept to help regulate your mind.

The mind is constantly streaming thoughts and making choices. When the mind begins to overexert is when you may start to feel anxious or have trouble sleeping. Just like anything else, the mind needs a break. When the balance between the three gunas is there, the mind will automatically take breaks or stay active as needed. The three gunas are responsible within the mind to bring about balance. Sattva would be thinking as necessary, rajas is to stay on track and stop the mind from wandering off onto tangent thoughts, and tamas is to stop thinking and quiet the mind. Most meditation or relaxation techniques are created with the purpose to balance the three gunas.

If the light was always green, the mind would keep going constantly, to the point where you would reach your destination but would still keep driving because there is no ability to slow down or switch off. Think of it as if your car brakes failed, and you could not stop. That is why rajas and tamas are important qualities to have. Of course, the opposite could happen in that you constantly stay on a red light, which is often when you feel lethargic or depressed. Excess rajas is often when you feel lost or confused and are not sure in which direction to go. In an imbalanced state of mind, the three gunas work in extremes. Yes, sattva, or purity, is also very important, but you still need all three.

Take a moment to sit and reflect. I would like you to take a deep breath in and reflect without judgement about where your mind feels it is at. You do not necessarily have to classify yourself as having a sattvic, rajasic, or tamasic mind. Rather, does your mind feel overactive, stable, confused, calm, or depressed? Anything that you feel is completely fine. We are not here to judge. Simply be with your thoughts because including your mind in how you make your choices is very important for your mental health. We often associate health with body only, but your mind and spirit play equal roles. Take a few minutes and write down how your mind is feeling.

Body is often more relatable when it comes to overall health and well-being. Any physical sign or symptom is associated with bodily health. When anyone falls ill, even if it's just a cold, you often immediately think of how your body feels: "My body is achy. I feel really cold." The body is what we use physically the most, and it can be seen more tangibly. The body runs all the physical functions such as digestion, metabolism, circulation, immunity response, the nervous system, and so much more. The bodily systems can be seen from the inside and outside with the help of modern technology.

The spirit has more of a deeper meaning. Your internal spirit is where your core values are held. This is who you are at your essence. Although some people associate the spirit with religion or spirituality, this does not have to be the case. The spirit is left for you to interpret as to what it means for you. The spirit is also what ties together the mind and the body. They have their separate functions, but they work together at the same time. In terms of the spirit, health is often correlated with your own inner sense of joy, confidence, beliefs, and the strength you have that comes from within. These beliefs and values you hold will often reflect within your physical, mental, and emotional health.[12]

If you integrate the mind, body, and spirit, it becomes easier to get healthy and feel your best. Ayurveda is wonderful in connecting the three. As with the three gunas for the mental qualities, Ayurveda educates how you can use various tools or modalities that support each of the three areas of the mind, body, and spirit individually and as a whole. The mind can be supported through the acts of meditation and mindfulness. The body is supported through food and routine, which includes activities. Spirit is held up through finding happiness and purpose in life. Engaging all three in a balanced way at any point will help you live in the present moment and not get caught up in the past or the future. Mindful eating is an excellent practice that engages the mind, body, and spirit.

To practice mindful eating, you must sit down to eat in a quiet and settled environment that is free from distractions. As you have your plate in front of you, your full attention should be place upon your meal. Then as you begin to eat, take the time to chew your food and assess it to taste all the flavours within your meal. Ask yourself how the food makes you feel. What flavours do you notice? Are you eating too quickly or too slowly? Then as you chew and swallow, pay attention to how you feel as the food begins to settle in your stomach. Continue to eat this way. Be mindful of how much you are putting into your mouth, how your mouth feels, and any sensations you may feel in your body as you chew and swallow. This will also allow you to have more awareness of when you are full as opposed to feeling stuffed. The practice of mindful eating will help you gain a better understanding of how different foods make you feel and what your own individual capacity is for how much food you can actually eat.

Simply knowing the roles and functions of each of the mind, body, and spirit allows for greater awareness of the self. Your overall health is dependent on you being self-aware and checking in with yourself. For example, it is only when you begin to have chronic acid reflux that you decide to take action and do something about making yourself feel better. Likewise, when it comes to being self-referral, you also want to be able to check in with yourself in terms of mind and spirit to recognise when something is off balance. Even with the body, it is best to not wait until the problem gets worse; rather, you should address your wellness challenges at the surface when they first arise.

The truth is one without the other will leave you feeling incomplete. A healthy body without a healthy mind can lead to mental health challenges. For example, physically you may feel in excellent shape; you exercise and eat well. However, you do very little to take care of your stress, or you seldom express your emotions. This can lead to anxiety, depression, sadness, and even loneliness or isolated. Opposite that, a healthy mind without a healthy body can lead to more physical illnesses. I used to run specific courses for diabetics to help them manage their type 2 diabetes. At the first introductory meeting, I met the students who were considering signing up for the programme. Some of them were completely happy to manage their diabetes with medication only, with no regard to their long-term physical health. For them, in the moment, they feel that medication helps them control their blood sugar levels without having to change the way they live, so this makes them happy and mentally causes no stress or anxiety. However, when diabetics manage their blood sugar levels with medication alone and without considering their dietary or lifestyle needs, then they will eventually fall physically ill. Therefore, it is possible to be completely content and have balanced mental health, but to suffer physically.

A healthy mind and a healthy body combo is also very likely. But without a healthy spirit, you may end up feeling that you lack meaning or purpose in life. You may not feel overall satisfaction with life, and you may not feel as happy as maybe you once did. Feelings such as these are often associated with depression. With the right treatment, including talk therapy, this can be overcome so that your spirit feels nourished and balanced. Spirit is about finding the truth of who you are, what you enjoy doing, and where your core values lie. An example is that you have an excellent job and a good family, but you still feel like something is missing. You may feel that you need more of a purpose. Everything may look good on paper, but you need more meaning to your life. This is where you need to explore finding yourself and developing the spirit side of your health.

All of this means that there is more to healthy living than diet and exercise. You must find joy and a reason to be happy. If it's not fun and you have no reason, then the changes will not last. You must be able to answer, "Why do you want to be healthy? Why are you interested in healthy living?" I always ask all my clients what their top five health goals are. The reason being that even if you do not have symptoms, you need a reason to make healthy changes. Without a reason that is motivating enough, you will not be able to create sustainable new habits.

Habits take time to form and establish. A common quote is, "There is no diet that will do what healthy eating does." I have a client who has recently lost ten kilogrammes in the last six months, and his friends constantly ask him, "Which diet are you on?" He responds, "I am not on any diet but rather have created new dietary and lifestyle habits." He feels better in himself and is able to find more joy in all he does because he consistently has more energy. This is why the holistic approach works. Diets do not give joy in the long run, and exercise may not necessarily be fun, but it is important that whatever you do for your mental and physical health, you incorporate your spirit into it. Finding happiness is truly an inside job. True happiness comes from within you and cannot be found in temporary changes. Everything you do must bring you joy and meaning.

When it comes to your health, you can make all the changes physically, but you must also address your mind and spirit. With many of my diabetic clients, I have seen that high stress levels can cause blood sugar fluctuations. High stress can affect your other hormones as well such as your adrenaline and cortisol levels, which triggers your "fight or flight" response. Stress can be felt physically but can also be felt within the mind and spirit.

In the last few decades, there has been a new movement that has formed known as consciousness-based health care. This movement is commonly associated with a modern branch of Ayurveda known as Maharishi Ayurveda. Maharishi Ayurveda is a revival of authentic Ayurvedic knowledge.[13] The founding team states that the knowledge of Ayurveda has become diluted over the decades and has lost its purity and authenticity. Maharishi Mahesh Yogi, also the founder of transcendental meditation, has revived the knowledge of Ayurveda and classified it as Maharishi Ayurveda. I have seen the difference in my time spent in India and during my clinical practice of Ayurveda and Maharishi Ayurveda. The main difference is that Maharishi Ayurveda makes it a point to integrate the mind, body, and spirit, whereas modern Ayurveda practitioners address the body primarily, then the mind only if they must.

I have seen many modern Ayurveda practitioners treat their clients only on the level of physical symptoms. They spend no more than five to ten minutes with their patients before recommending herbs and moving on to their next patient. Ayurveda does have an entire branch of herbs or medicine, but it is not the only area of expertise of Ayurvedic medicine. The body should always be treated as a whole and not just within its parts. Within the essence of Ayurveda is trying to find the root cause of the imbalance and working within the mind, body, and spirit to find balance and health.

Consciousness is such a vast term with multiple meanings. However, I am not referring here to the mental status of alertness. According to Maharishi Ayurveda, "Consciousness is that which is most intimate to our experience—that which lies beneath thought and feeling. It is awareness itself, the experiencer."[14] Consciousness is the principle that unifies the mind, body, and spirit and is the inner intelligence that your body has. Think of it this way: your body is so intelligent that it does many functions without you having to do anything, such as the way the heart beats on its own, or how your liver filters toxins. Understanding the unifying force of consciousness helps you make choices that are in line with the needs of your mind, body, and spirit. Remember that the reason you struggle is because you are feeling out of balance. Perfect health means you are feeling balanced within your mind, body, and spirit, and therefore the inner intelligence or consciousness is lively. As a result, you are able to engage in self-referral or be established in self-awareness so that you know when you are feeling balanced and imbalanced.

YOU CAN FEEL HEALTHY AGAIN BY FOLLOWING THE PRINCIPLES OF AYURVEDA

At its core, Ayurveda has never been about treating the disease, but initially it had its focus on the prevention of disease. It is estimated that Ayurveda was founded around the sixth century BCE,[15] which dates further back than Hippocrates. Now, Hippocrates also emphasised that prevention is preferable to cure. Prevention is in fact easier to manage than it is to cure or treat a disease or imbalance. For example, many modern-day diseases such as heart disease and type 2 diabetes can be prevented by adapting a healthy diet and lifestyle. Prevention also means that you do not have to worry about ill health, taking medication, the side effects of medication, your blood test results, or any other additional health screenings and checks in relation to an ongoing condition.

Some diseases cannot be prevented, but in most cases, you can choose how you take care of yourself when being treated. I have a client, Naomi, who was diagnosed with multiple sclerosis back in 2016, and she was forty-six at the time. As soon as she was diagnosed, she began her research, educated herself, and looked for alternative treatments. Within weeks of being diagnosed, she came to me to be her nutritionist, and thus began our journey of working together. I am able to offer her the integrative approach to nutrition, and that was what appealed to her the most. We improved her diet, addressed her lifestyle, and ensured that she was on the correct supplements along with managing her stress. She even began to attend my yoga classes. Naomi took her health into her own hands and has stayed in remission all these years due to her commitment to taking care of her health.

To prevent disease means to be proactive about your own health. You must be your own advocate and listen to your body and its needs. You cannot put off till tomorrow what can be done today about your health. "Oh, I will drink more water tomorrow" will not help your body to stay hydrated today. Ayurveda does place a heavy emphasis on diet and what you eat, but it also focuses on how there are numerous other influences to your overall health. Some are within your control, and others, such as the seasons, are out of your control. Winter months are known to have a great number of colds and flus, but Ayurveda is prepared for that as well. Ayurveda has a very unique approach that teaches everyone how to be ready for the unexpected and to keep your health balanced despite external influences.

Maharishi Mahesh Yogi stated, "Diet is anything that is taken in from any field of perception, through any sense of perception, any mode of mind, and any mode of intellect."[16] This means that diet is not just your food but also includes all experiences. It is a completely true point in that any experience you have must be processed in some way, shape, or form by your mind, body, and spirit. Food is a concrete example of how your body will digest the food. Your mind will also make it a point to remember it, and your spirit will recognise whether or not that piece of food brought you any joy or meaning. Similarly, all other experiences are processed. Oftentimes after you have a heated conversation with someone, you will reflect back and say to yourself, "This particular experience did not sit well with me." Although physically you ate nothing, your mind and spirit are processing the interaction, and your stomach or gut is having to deal with it as well.

The basic foundation of Ayurveda rests upon the five elements, or Pancha Mahabhutas. These five elements are akasha (space or ether), vayu (air), agni (fire), jal (water), and prithvi (earth). All these elements are found in the environment and within the human body. An example of each of these within the human physiology is that the emptiness or gap between bones or around joints is space, oxygen within the lungs is air, digestion and its acids are fire, blood is water, and tissues are earth. The way the elements work together is where Ayurveda gives us the teachings and shows us how well we are connected internally and externally.

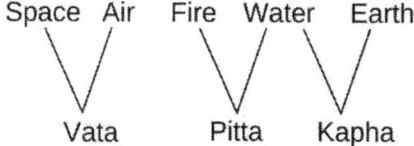

The elements come dynamically together to form what are known as the doshas, or energies. There are three doshas of vata, pitta, and kapha. Vata is comprised of air and space, pitta is made from fire and water, and kapha consists of water and earth. The elements do not work on their own but they work together. When the elements come together, each dosha has its primary qualities, which are as follows.

> Vata: dry, rough, light, moving, changing, abundant, cold, coarse, brittle, nonsticky

> Pitta: slightly oily, hot, warm, sharp, liquid, flowing, sour, pungent

> Kapha: heavy, cold, soft, oily, sweet, stable, steady, sticky

These qualities can be seen everywhere. Being of air and space, it makes sense that vata is vast and constantly changing. The wind of vata brings the qualities of dryness and coarseness. Pitta, being of fire and water, would naturally make it on the warmer side, sharp and fluid-like. When you put water and earth together, kapha brings about heaviness, stability, and sticky, and it is also quite cool. Vata, pitta, and kapha can be seen functioning within the human physiology as well as in the environment around us. Along with the qualities, each of the doshas has its own functions.

Vata controls all the movement, communication, and transformation functions within the body. This includes the nervous system, circulatory system, colon, bladder, and kidneys, as well as the movement of arms and legs. Vata also plays a strong role with levels of enthusiasm; breathing; elimination of urine, sweat, and faeces; development as you grow and age; and any other movement-related functioning of the body such as blinking of the eyes. In a balanced state, vata people have a tendency to be thin or lighter in weight, be prone to dry skin, be mentally and physically active, have irregular appetite and digestion, be alert, talk quickly, be creative, and be enthusiastic in all that they do.

Pitta's main functions include digestion, metabolism, and transformation. The key areas in which pitta operates is the digestive system, small intestine, blood, and eyes. Other areas of function include the entire digestive process, sight, thirst, hunger, lustre of skin, and the intellect. Pitta plays a crucial role in not only digesting food but also in metabolising and absorbing the nutrients that you consume. In addition, pitta is also what drives passion and gives a person motivation to get things done. It also resides in both the emotional and physical heart. Pitta people are often of medium built and weight, have think and silky hair, have good quality of sleep, have sharp intellects, and are courageous, organised, and focused.

Kapha has its main functions in the structure, cohesion, and lubrication of the body. Kapha holds together the tissues, joints, neck, chest, and head, to name a few. By and large, kapha upholds the entire body and gives you the structure and foundation you have. Some of its other functions include strength, levels of patience, and potency. Kapha people are well built and tend to be on the heavier side. They have soft and oily skin, thick and wavy hair, and large and soft eyes. They have a slow digestion and metabolism, sleep soundly, and have a lasting memory. They are very sweet, affectionate, generous people who are quick to forgive.

There is also a lot of crossover with the doshas because none of their functions are exclusive to them. For example, vata controls speech, but pitta governs the emotions behind the speech, and kapha supports the structure of the tongue and throat so that the speech can come out. This is how the mind, body, and spirit are represented within the doshas. Vata is the mind, pitta is the spirit, and kapha is the body. Vata also controls prana, or the breath, which is the life force. Without prana, there is no life, which means there is no body or spirit either. Pitta is considered to be the spirit as emotions rise from the heart. This fiery dosha controls passion and determination, which is necessary for a healthy spirit. Kapha is structure and therefore represents the body. There is an overlap between these, but this is probably one of the most concrete ways to demonstrate how intimately the mind, body, and spirit are connected.

Each dosha, when imbalanced, can give rise to some specific symptoms that help you identify which doshas need to be pacified or balanced. They are as follows.

Vata: dry or rough skin, constipation, general fatigue, tension headaches, intolerance of cold, degenerative arthritis, underweight, anxiety, excessive thoughts or thinking, worrying in excess, thinning or brittleness of hair, difficulty falling asleep or insomnia, irregular digestion

Pitta: rashes, acne, psoriasis, inflammatory skin diseases, inflammatory bowel diseases, visual problems, heartburn, peptic ulcers, excessive body heat, premature greying of hair, premature balding, hostility, irritability, anger, fast metabolism

Kapha: oily skin, excessive sleep, lethargy, mental dullness, slow digestion, sinus congestion, nasal allergies, asthma, cysts and other growths, obesity, greedy, slow to start, possessiveness, depression, sad/depressed mood

Ayurveda clearly states, "Vata, Pitta, and Kapha are the three fundamental principles governing physiological processes. When in balance, they maintain the body in good health, when out of balance, they are the three basic causes of imbalance, disturbance, and disease in the body."[17] To be proactive about your health, it is important to know how your doshas are feeling and know which are balanced and which are out of balance. Those who are well versed in Ayurveda will automatically know which factors are disturbing the doshas and the steps to take care of it. The next couple of chapters will help you gain a much more thorough understanding of the doshas, how they influence you, how to identify which doshas need to be balanced, and the actions that you need to take.

Vaidyas (doctors of Ayurveda) or qualified Ayurvedic health practitioners are the best people to give you a thorough assessment of the doshas. They will use a variety of techniques ranging from questions and answers to health questionnaires and pulse diagnosis. If meeting the client in person, I use all three, but if the consultation takes place remotely, then pulse diagnosis is not feasible. When doshas are assessed, the bigger picture as well as the parts of the picture need to be thoroughly analysed. Knowing symptoms is important, but the goal of any Ayurvedic practitioner is to find the root cause of the imbalance. Treating the symptoms is merely a topical approach. The cause needs to be found and treated at the root of the imbalance. What caused the problem to begin with? Oftentimes the root cause cannot be specifically identified, and that is where the doshas play a larger role. Through a thorough dosha assessment, it can be identified which doshas are the most imbalanced and which dosha is causing the other doshas to go off course. The ultimate goal is to balance the doshas so that you are in your natural state.

With dosha assessments, there is a difference between balanced and imbalanced doshas and how they are truly assessed. When you take a dosha quiz, which you are about to do shortly, or when an Ayurvedic practitioner gives you your dosha assessment, this is known as your vikriti, or current state of health. It does not necessarily identify who you are at the core. Your doshic balance at the core is known as prakriti, and this is your natural constitution. Prakriti is who you are at the very root and where your natural tendencies lie.

Vikriti is your current imbalance, or rather current state of health, and it is over a result of multiple influences such as diet, lifestyle, sleep, and stress. This reflects in your pulse from months or even years' worth of imbalances. However, vikriti can also change quite quickly—for example, the sudden loss of a loved one, moving homes, or even travel can change your vikriti. More long-term changes are reflected primarily through dietary and lifestyle habits. Furthermore, the environment, such as the seasons, will also influence vikriti.

The purpose behind a dosha assessment is to know which doshas are balanced and which ones are not. This will allow for more specific advice regarding how to achieve balance. When consulting with a specialist about your doshas, this will also help them assess which doshas were affected at the root cause so you can heal from inside out. As you work to balance the doshas, your prakriti will become more apparent, and your natural state will be able to shine. Ultimately, you want the vikriti to be in alignment with the prakriti. It is also important to note that you do not want to get lost in trying to determine your prakriti because this is best done by working with a specialist. The real secret is that you use your current state of healthy to restore balance.

The prakriti will eventually reveal itself, but for now it is best to live in the moment and work with what you know. When you take the dosha quiz below, answer honestly so that you can determine your vikriti.

For this dosha assessment, circle or check your answer based upon how you have been feeling in the last couple of weeks. Try not to think too far back because it may skew your results. The vikriti should be based upon how you are feeling at the moment, however you can include symptoms that you experience on a regular basis within the last couple of weeks. Each section has its own further set of instructions.

Section 1: Check all that apply. Circle or check all the symptoms that you have

Category A	Category B	Category C
Insomnia	Diarrhoea	Congestion
Gas	Loose stools	Food or Respiratory Allergies
Bloating	Nausea	Oedema/water retention
Constipation	Migraines	Heaviness
Muscle twitching, cramping, numbness, or weakness	Vomiting	Dullness
Joint pain/joint cracking	Skin rashes	Dull pain
Stiffness	Acne	Cold, clammy hands
Moving pain	Bruising	Difficulty sweating
Dry cough	Excess thirst	Frequent urination
Cold extremities	Burning, sharp pain	Excess oily skin
Dry skin	Excess body heat	Excess sleep
Restlessness	Interrupted sleep/ trouble staying asleep	Depression

Category A	Category B	Category C
Worry	Judgemental/Critical	Greed
Fear	Anger	Attachment
Anxiety	Feeling envious	Mental lethargy

Section 2: Only select one answer from each row. If you feel that more than one applies, select the one that is more applicable.

	Category A	Category B	Category C
Body Frame	Slim	Medium	Large
Body Weight	Low	Medium	Overweight
Chin	Thin, angular	Tapering	Rounded (double)
Eyes	Small, sunken	Sharp, bright	Big, beautiful
Nose	Uneven (angled)	Long and pointed	Short, rounded (button nose)
Lips	Dry, cracked	Red, inflamed	Smooth, oily
Skin	Dry, thin, cold	Smooth, oily, warm	Thick, oily, cool
Hair	Dry, brittle, thin	Straight, oily, greyness, or balding	Thick, curly, oily
Nails	Dry, rough, brittle	Sharp, flexible, lustrous	Thick, oily, smooth
Hips	Slender, thin	Moderate	Heavy, big
Joints	Cold, cracking	Moderate	Large, lubricated
Appetite	Irregular	Strong, unbearable	Slow, but steady
Digestion	Irregular, gassy at times	Quick, burning sensation	Slow, feel heavy
Thirst levels	Vary	Excessive	Sparse
Elimination	Constipation	Loose	Sluggish
Physical	Hyperactive	Moderate	Slow

	Category A	Category B	Category C
Mental	Overactive mind	Sharp intellect	Takes time to process
Emotions	Anxiety, fear, uncertainty	Anger, hate, jealousy	Calm, greedy, Attachment
Response	Quick and impulsive	Fast and passionate	Slow and precise
Memory	Recent good, history poor	Precise	Slow and sustained
Sleep	Sleeplessness, trouble falling asleep	Little but sound	Deep and can sleep anytime anywhere
Speech	Fast and mumbled	Sharp and loud	Slow but steady
Temperament	Moody	Volatile	Soft-spoken
Appearance	Thin, bony	Medium, intense	Large, sluggish
Energy levels	Hyperactive	Intense	Low
Total from Sections 1 and 2:			

Be sure to tally up the total number that you checked or marked off for each column. Once you have your total numbers for each column, proceed to determine what your results mean.

Category A is vata
Category B is pitta
Category C is kapha

Whichever column has the most checked off is the strongest dosha at the moment and therefore signifies your vikriti or current state of health. It is also possible to have the same number in two or all three columns. For example, if you have a total of fourteen for both categories A and B, this means that you are vata-pitta. There are seven different dosha combinations that can come about from this assessment.

vata
pitta
kapha
vata-pitta
vata-kapha
pitta-kapha
vata-pitta-kapha

Now that you are aware of your state of health, as you continue to read the book, you will want to focus on the factors that will help balance your doshas. Some of the recommendations will help all doshas regardless of what your score was, but others are more specific. In the cases where more than one dosha came out on top, you want to favour the one that is first. For example, in vata-pitta, favour balancing vata first. For pitta-kapha, primarily focus on balancing pitta first. The reason is that the doshas move in order. Vata is known as the king dosha, and it leads the way. The air and space elements of vata is what helps keep the flow and the other doshas moving.

In its main text, *Charaka Samhita*, Ayurveda states, "Without a proper diet, herbs are of no use. With a proper diet, herbs are of no need."[18] Although Ayurveda has herbal remedies, this statement essentially means that your diet will play a greater role in your health than anything else. Keep in mind that your lifestyle and actions are also a part of your diet. As we move forward from here, we will focus on the main areas of how Ayurveda can help you through prevention of disease and how your choices influence your health.

Knowing your vikriti or current state of health also helps to identify which health problems you want to try and avoid. Referring back to the list of possible conditions, if you are a pitta vikriti, you now know that you are more susceptible to developing skin conditions. Therefore skin should be well taken care of, and you also want to apply pitta-pacifying measures that you will soon learn so that pitta can express itself in a balanced state. This is where you want to focus on yourself and apply all that you have learned through the self-awareness exercises.

Each dosha type has its own personality type that goes with it. When imbalanced, a vata person can often be overwhelmed with the feelings of fear, grief, worry, anxiety, and restlessness. However, in general, vata people are also very active both mentally and physically. They are creative, can be unorganised, and are generally late to appointments. They are always "running behind schedule". Their memories are erratic, and decision-making is impulsive.

Pitta imbalances often result in anger, hatred, jealousy, and passion. However, when in balance they are intelligent, perfectionists, competitive, organised, and efficient. They are excellent leaders but can also be anxious and have a fear of failure. Pitta people are passionate people and will always go above and beyond the call of duty.

Kapha types, when imbalanced, are generally filled with greed, attachment, dullness, and being slow. However, when balanced, they are the opposite of vata people. They talk and move more slowly because they like steadiness and stability. They are always on time, if not early, and they love to follow rules but are also calm and easy-going. They are excellent friends because they are loyal, forgiving, affectionate, and dependable. This also means that kapha people are often resistant to change and can be stubborn.

Keep in mind that these are generalisations, and qualities can vary from person to person. You may find that you resonate with just one dosha, two, or even all three dosha personality types. This is a part of getting to know yourself as you begin to take action steps to find balance.

You do not have to do everything. This is the largest mistake people make when trying to apply the principles of Ayurveda into their life. Ayurveda has never stated that you must follow every principle it lays out; rather, it is about prioritising. Just like when we discussed self-care and prioritising your needs, you must set realistic expectations when applying what you are learning. If you set the bar too high or try to do too much in one go, then the changes will not have a lasting impact. Trust me on this. With all my clients, I have them start with small changes and gradually work their way up. The goal is to not have temporary fixes but to have lasting changes that have a healthy impact on your life. Therefore, promise me that you will not set unrealistic expectations and that you shall prioritise and start with what is most important. Then you can gradually add in more as needed.

When working with my clients, I use little to no supplementation because my working philosophy is what the *Charaka Samhita* stated. With that said, I do recommend supplements when needed to provide the additional support or boost, but this is often short-term. No supplement will accomplish what real food is meant to do. This is also why the "real food" or "clean eating" movement has gained so much traction. Real, wholesome food is filled with nutritious goodness, fibre, and the nutrients you eat in a natural state are more easily absorbable than what you take in the form of a supplement.[19]

In addition to eating real food, Ayurveda also emphasises following an ideal daily routine known as dinacharya. The recommended daily routine follows the dosha clock. This dosha clock outlines the times of day in which vata, pitta, and kapha are energetically the strongest within the environment thus having a greater influence on how you feel. As you can see from the clock, the vata dosha is dominant between the hours of two to six both mornings and afternoons, kapha is strongest between six and ten both mornings and evenings, and pitta is strongest between ten and two both midday and night. Regardless of what your vikriti is, by following the suggested activities during the specific times of the day, it can have a balancing effect on all your doshas.

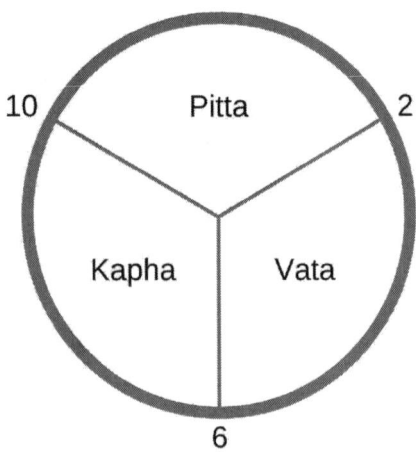

Beginning with the morning, it is best to rise before 6.00 a.m. so that you can have the vata energy with you throughout the day. Vata is all about movement, and if you rise with it, then you are likely to have more energy throughout the day. Upon waking up, evacuate your bowels and bladder, followed by brushing your teeth, scraping your tongue, and gargling with oil. Next, do daily abhyanga, which is a self-oil massage. If you do not have time to massage your entire body, then it is best to focus on massaging your head, body, and soles of feet. Be careful not to slip on the oil. While you allow the oil to seep into your skin, ideally leaving on for about twenty minutes, this is a great time to relax and do some reading or breathing exercises. It is also a good time to enjoy a cup of hot water with lemon (or plain warm water if you are a pitta type). Next up is taking a bath or shower, after which you put on clean and comfortable clothes to suit the season and activity. Then it is best to do your morning yoga practice, if you have one. After that is the best time to have a light breakfast.

This is a lot to incorporate to your morning routine, especially if you are already short on time. Therefore, be sure to prioritise. Start by picking one or two items to focus on from the list above and then slowly add more when it is possible. Ayurveda suggests that the most important is to rise before kapha time sets in, because once kapha time of the day starts and you wake up with that, then you are likely to have a more lethargic or less focused of day. Once you are in kapha time of the day, this is the best time of the day to do some exercise. Activity is a great way to counter the excess effects of kapha and boost energy levels.

As you continue through your morning routine, continue to be active and completing your tasks at hand. Once you hit the pitta time of the day, this is when digestion is strongest. This is why lunch should be the largest meal of the day, because your body will more easily be able to digest and metabolise the food you eat slightly. After lunch, it is best to rest for a short time to allow the digestive process to continue. Then it is all about continuing your day.

Once you hit the vata period in the evening, it is time for dinner ensuring the food you eat is in accordance with your dosha and taking into account the season along with any other factors, such as food intolerances. After dinner is a nice time to take a short ten- to fifteen-minute walk. Then it is best to engage in pleasant and relaxing activity before going to bed by 10 p.m. To improve quality of sleep, it is recommended that you refrain from using your phone and tablets and watching television because the light sends the wrong signal and may prevent melatonin from being released, thereby delaying the onset of sleep.[20] The reason why Ayurveda recommends going to sleep before 10.00 a.m. is once pitta time starts, that is when you will experience your "second wind" and therefore get a slight energy boost. It makes it harder to fall asleep during this time.

Once your head hits the pillow, ideally you should be able to stay asleep until it is time to wake up. Depending on your dosha, you may need more or less sleep. Vata and pitta people can get by with less sleep, but kapha people definitely need their sleep. Either way, regardless of which dosha you are, it is important to establish regular sleep and wake times that are consistent throughout the week. This means that you should sleep and rise at the same time on the weekdays and weekends. It is better for your internal clock, which controls your circadian rhythms, that you establish a routine. It may feel hard at first, but your mind, body, and spirit will thank you for it.

EAT ACCORDING TO YOUR BODY TYPE AND DOSHA

One of the biggest mistakes people make when choosing a new approach is that they follow the herd and do the same as everybody else. That is why fad diets become so popular: because people automatically assume that if something worked for somebody else, then it will naturally work for them too. But that is not true. As the classic saying goes, one man's medicine is another man's poison. Any approach or model you take on should recognise that you are an individual who is different from the billions of other people in this world. You have different life experiences, and your health situation is different. I have said this before, and I will say it again: no two clients of mine are on the same dietary or lifestyle plan. Each person is different, so how can the exact same approach work for everybody? Sure, it may appear that the same approach works, but the truth of the matter is that it does not.

The first step to customisation of a plan is your dietary choices. If you eat according to your dosha, you will feel your best, and that will help you achieve a balanced state of health. There are six tastes in Ayurveda: sweet, sour, salty, pungent, bitter, and astringent. The tastes are made from the five elements of space, air, fire, water, and earth. Each taste is made from two of the elements, which are as follows.

Sweet: water and earth
Sour: fire and earth
Salty: fire and water
Pungent: air and fire
Bitter: space and air
Astringent: air and earth

Each taste plays a role in whether it increases or decreases the doshas. As you can see from the following chart, vata is decreased or pacified by favouring the sweet, sour, and salty tastes. Pitta is balanced or pacified by having the sweet, bitter, and astringent tastes. Kapha is pacified or restored by favouring the pungent, bitter, and astringent tastes. Although these are the tastes that you want to favour, it is important to have all six tastes for your main meals throughout the day. The six tastes each have a function or role they play, especially when it comes to digestion and overall health. Therefore it is about finding the right balance within your meals. Following the principles of the six tastes will naturally create more balanced meals and will also eliminate any food cravings, along with providing satiety or sense of comfort after each meal.

	Vata	Pitta	Kapha
Sweet	Decrease	Decrease	Increase
Sour	Decrease	Increase	Increase
Salty	Decrease	Increase	Increase
Pungent	Increase	Increase	Decrease
Bitter	Increase	Decrease	Decrease
Astringent	Increase	Decrease	Decrease

The sweet taste promotes strength, is good for the throat, and helps heal fractures. It is nourishing, helps many vital functions, and is great for complexion, hair, and the sensory organs. Although it is heavy for digestion, it generally provides the feeling of satisfaction or pleasantness to the sensory organs. When consumed in excess, it can cause tumours, obesity, and diabetes. Keep in mind that the sweet taste will increase kapha but decrease vata and pitta. Some examples of sweet taste are grains such as wheat, rice, and barley; pulses; lentils; milk; cream; butter; sweet fruits such as dates, figs, coconut, and mango; cooked vegetables such as potato, carrot, and cauliflower; and of course sugar.

The sour taste makes the mouth water, and its properties are light, oily, and hot. Therefore the sour taste increases pitta and kapha, meaning vata is decreased. Sour taste is great for stimulating the taste buds, it increases appetite, and it is good for the heart. Excess intake can lead to acidity, heartburn, gastritis, swelling, itching, trouble with eyesight, and fever. Some examples of sour tastes are sour fruits such as lemon, oranges, and pineapples; sour milk products such as yogurt, cheese, and sour cream; fermented substances such as wine, vinegar, and soy sauce; and carbonated beverages.

The salty taste decreases vata but increases pitta and kapha. The salty taste increases salivation and has the qualities of heaviness and warmth. It is also good for digestion and clears up any obstruction in the channels of circulation. Excessive salt intake can lead to high blood pressure, kidney disease, excessive thirst, skin disease, and even stroke. Salt is needed in all diets, but in small amounts. In order to get the salty taste in your diet, you must add a type of salt to your food, even if it is a minute amount.

The pungent taste is a sharp taste and is most often associated with spicy flavours. Pungent taste will decrease kapha because it has a stimulating and sharp effect, which means that it will increase vata and pitta. The pungent taste is good for digestion and throat problems, and it may help alleviate constipation. When used in excess, it can lead to fainting, tremors, heartburn, and diarrhoea, and aggravate allergic reactions. The pungent taste is found in spices, such as chilli powder, black pepper, mustard seeds, ginger, cardamom, garlic, turmeric, cinnamon, oregano, and mint. Raw vegetables such as onion and cauliflower are also pungent in taste.

The bitter taste will increase vata but decrease pitta and kapha. The bitter taste is light, dry, and cold, which helps to cleanse the palette and has an overall detoxing effect on the body; it also helps to prevent blood-related disorders. However, when consumed in excess, the bitter taste can weaken the tissues of the body and reduce overall strength. The bitter taste is found in most green vegetables, especially leafy greens such as spinach and cabbage. Fruits such as olives and grapefruits and spices such as fenugreek and turmeric are also bitter in taste.

The astringent taste is heavy, dry, and cold. It will increase vata and decrease pitta and kapha. Astringent taste cleanses the blood and skin and also dries up excess moisture and fat in the body. Excessive intake can slow down digestion and cause flatulence, chest pain, excessive thirst, and constipation. Some examples of the astringent taste are turmeric, honey, walnuts, hazelnuts, pulses, beans, vegetables such as sprouts and lettuce, and fruits such as pomegranates, berries, and most unripe fruits.

Most foods and spices have more than one taste, such as turmeric, which is pungent, bitter, and astringent. Therefore each food or spice will play multiple roles in the body. In the pages to follow, you will find a list of foods and spices to favour to pacify your predominant dosha based upon your vikriti from the quiz earlier. This list is not exhaustive. Favour as many of those foods and spices as you can the majority of the time, but do not be afraid to deviate slightly from the plan. Eating well is also about eating flexibly. Using the six tastes is a great way to adapt your diet to the needs of your body.

VATA PACIFYING DIET

General: Consume warm, unctuous, and nourishing foods with moderation in portion sizes. Avoid cold and dry foods. Avoid skipping meals or having too little of food.

Grains: whole wheat, couscous, amaranth, quinoa, rice, cooked oats

Legumes: yellow split mung beans, red lentils, mung dahl, tofu, toor dahl, urad dahl

Vegetables: zucchini (courgette), asparagus, carrot, beetroot, sweet potato, radish, pumpkin, celery, parsnip, tomato, artichoke, cucumber, yellow squash, okra, tender eggplant, turnips, rhubarb, yellow and orange capsicum peppers

Fruits: All ripe sweet, juicy fruits. Dried fruit is better soaked in water before eating. Grapes, banana, melon, plums, cherries, kiwi, peaches, apricots, mangos, papaya, pomegranate, sweet pineapple, avocado, sweet oranges, grapefruit, sweet clementines, raisins, dates, prunes, honeydew, sweet strawberries, sweet blackberries, sweet raspberries, coconuts, and figs. Apples and pears, but only if they are sweet and juicy.

Dairy: milk (boiled and served hot), butter, ghee, cream, yogurt, soft cheeses (such as ricotta, cottage cheese and cream cheese), paneer, sour cream

Nuts and Seeds: almonds, cashews, pistachios, walnuts, pecans, pine nuts, macadamia nuts, hazelnuts, sesame seeds, sunflower seeds, pumpkin seeds, poppy seeds

Oils: almond oil, avocado oil, castor oil, coconut oil, ghee, olive oil, sunflower oil, sesame oil

Meat: eggs, chicken, beef, salmon, white fish, duck

Spices and Herbs: cumin, ginger, mustard seeds, hing (asafoetida), cinnamon, cardamom, clove, anise, fennel, black pepper (small amounts), rock salt, lemon juice, tamarind, coriander leaves and seeds, saffron, vanilla, nutmeg, rosemary, thyme, lemongrass, oregano, and basil. All others in small amounts.

PITTA PACIFYING DIET

General: Favour cool and cooling foods, and ensure you stay hydrated and are eating sufficiently sized meals. Avoid hot, dry, and excessively light or too small portions of food.

Grains: wheat, rice, oats, barley, wild rice, buckwheat

Legumes: mung beans, green peas, garbanzo beans, kidney beans, white beans, brown lentils, yellow and green split peas, toor dahl (pigeon pea), soybeans, and all other lentils

Vegetables: courgette, fennel, corn, artichoke, asparagus, green beans, French beans, runner beans, white radish, spinach, watercress, white pumpkin, celery, bitter gourd, sweet potato, broccoli, cauliflower, cabbage, chard, kale, caper, green papaya, plantain, lettuce, cucumber, ginger, eggplant, bean sprouts, okra, potato

Fruits: grapes, raisin, pomegranate, tangerine, sweet mandarin, clementine, sweet tangerine, sweet pineapple, avocado, persimmon, apricot, honeydew melon, cantaloupe, watermelon, kiwi, figs, dates, coconut, banana, guava, apples, peaches, cherries, mango, sweet strawberries, sweet blueberries, sweet blackberries, sweet raspberries

Dairy Products: milk, cream, butter, ghee, kefir, cream cheese, soft cheese, paneer, sweet lassi

Nuts and Seeds: pumpkin seeds, poppy seeds, pine nuts, macadamia nuts, sunflower seeds, blanched almonds

Oils: ghee, olive oil, coconut oil

Spices and Herbs: coriander, saffron, cinnamon, vanilla, rock salt, rose water, fennel seeds, ginger, cumin seeds, parsley, mint, cardamom, fenugreek, dill, lemon grass, clove, anise

Meats: chicken, turkey, eggs, and other white meats. Red meats should be avoided.

KAPHA PACIFYING DIET

General: Favour warm foods and drinks that are full of flavour yet are light and easy to digest. Avoid unctuous, cold, heavy food in large quantities, and avoid eating at night.

Grains: corn, barley, millet, rye, buckwheat

Legumes: mung beans, green peas, chickpeas, kidney beans, brown and green lentils, yellow and green split peas, pigeon pea, black-eyed peas

Vegetables: carrot, artichoke, asparagus, runner beans, tomato, eggplant, radish, spinach, watercress, pumpkin, celery, broccoli, cauliflower, Brussels sprouts, cabbage, red cabbage, chard, kale, caper, all bell peppers, alfalfa sprouts, bean sprouts, green beans, bamboo shoots, lettuce, parsnips, potatoes (minimum), cucumber

Fruits: (Sweeter fruits in smaller amounts.) Pomegranates, grapefruit, persimmon, plum, prune, strawberry, blueberry, blackberry, raspberries, blackcurrant, cranberry, apples, pears, pineapple, cherry, peaches, apricots, kiwi, guava, passion fruit, figs, dates, and coconut.

Dairy: Ghee and low-fat dairy products. It is best to use natural dairy alternatives where available, such as hemp or almond milk.

Oils (in small amounts): olive oil, sunflower oil, and mustard oil

Nuts and Seeds: sunflower seeds, pumpkin seeds, almonds, walnuts

Spices and Herbs: ginger, cumin seeds, coriander seeds, cilantro, parsley, mint, fennel seeds, anise, clove, saffron, cardamom, cinnamon, caraway seeds, ajowan seeds, black pepper, rock salt (in small amounts), asafoetida, fenugreek, nutmeg, oregano, dill seed, rosemary, thyme, lemongrass, turmeric, vanilla, paprika, chilli powder, garlic

Keep in mind that keeping the digestive fire balanced is the most important. According to Ayurveda, the health of your digestive fire is of the utmost importance. Within the Ayurvedic texts, it states, "No dosha, dhatu (tissue), mala (waste), or organ can perform its physiological functions without Agni."[21] Agni is your digestive fire, and the main agni is found in the stomach. There are numerous agnis, but the jathara agni is the most important. There are four primary states of the Agni: sama, visham, tikshna, and mand. Sama agni is a balanced and healthy agni. Visham is a vata-imbalanced agni, tikshna is imbalanced due to pitta, and a mand agni is the result of excess kapha.

VATA DIGESTION

A visham agni is an irregular one because it moves and changes due to the elements of air and space within vata. Therefore a visham agni may result in the following:

- irregular appetite
- indigestion
- alternating between diarrhoea and constipation
- constipation
- gas
- bloating
- colic-type pain
- a feeling of heaviness after meals
- gurgling of the intestines
- dry skin and mouth
- insomnia
- muscle spasms
- cracking and popping joints
- aches and pains
- deep-seated fears
- insecurity
- anxiety
- excessive craving of meats

A visham agni needs to be grounded, and a form of regularity or consistency needs to be established. Because metabolism is irregular, if you have a visham agni, sometimes you may feel fine, and other times you will have some of the symptoms listed earlier. Some days you feel well, and other days you do not. Vata imbalances are difficult to identify because the irregularity makes it difficult to pin down.

PITTA DIGESTION

A tikshna agni is the digestive fire that is fuelled by pitta. The fire and water elements make this fire very hot, and it is considered to be an overactive metabolism. Some of the signs of an overactive metabolism include the following.

- strong appetite
- must eat on time
- Iiritable if meals are missed
- hyperacidity
- heartburn
- acidic saliva
- nausea
- vomiting
- loose stools
- diarrhoea
- fever
- irritability
- aggressiveness
- desire to overcontrol
- gastritis
- colitis
- hives
- rashes
- acne
- other inflammatory skin conditions

Although having an extremely strong digestion sounds look a good thing, from the list of signs, you can see that it has its downfall too. Having an overactive metabolism means that your digestive system does not get the chance to absorb all the nutrients because food gets pushed through your system too quickly. This can lead to nutrient deficiencies and other problems such as premature greying or loss of hair.

KAPHA DIGESTION

A mand agni is a result of a kapha imbalance and results in a slow metabolism. Some of its signs and symptoms are as follows.

- poor appetite
- sluggish digestion
- heaviness in the stomach
- congestion
- cough
- nausea
- bloating
- lethargy
- excessive sleep
- cold clammy skin
- underactive thyroid
- overweight or obesity
- oedema
- generalised weakness
- hypertension
- attachment
- greed
- possessiveness
- depression
- lack of motivation

As you can see, a mand agni is one that slows down the digestion. One finds it hard to digest and break down food, which means that the body finds it hard to metabolise and absorb nutrients. With a kapha-influenced agni, you may often feel slow, lethargic, and heavy. It does not mean that you will gain weight, but it does mean that you may find it difficult to build muscle, and you cannot eat much without feeling overly stuffed.

BALANCED AND HEALTHY DIGESTION

Once you are familiar with the vata, pitta, and kapha associated agnis, there is still one more type of agni, known as sama agni, which is a balanced digestive fire. The goal of following an Ayurvedic diet and lifestyle is to ultimately achieve a state of balanced health, which can only happen once your agni is balanced. Here are the sings of a sama agni.

- normal levels of hunger and thirst
- subjective feeling of lightness in the stomach
- clean tongue, no coating on tongue when waking up
- good sense of taste
- alertness
- regular and well-formed bowel movements
- no constipation or diarrhoea
- good digestion and assimilation and absorption of nutrients
- healthy colour and complexion
- courage and confidence
- joy, cheerfulness, contentment
- mental clarity and wholeness
- enthusiasm
- well-nourished tissues
- intelligence
- patience
- healthy glow and lustre
- healthy immune system
- prana (breath) circulates freely
- enhanced longevity/lifespan
- vitality
- strength
- stamina
- balanced outlook

A balanced and healthy digestion leads to the production of ojas. Ojas represents your immune system, and in Ayurveda, it is the finest product of the material creation and is the junction point between consciousness and matter. This means that ojas is as much consciousness as it is matter. According to the texts of Ayurveda, ojas smells like roasted rice, is sweet to taste like honey, and is yellowish-white in colour. Because it is the finest product of digestion, it sustains all the dhatus (tissues), strengthens the immune system, and produces a feeling of happiness.

When ojas is lively, it is a symbol of good health and vitality. This is why having a healthy digestion is so important in Ayurveda. As mentioned before, prevention is key, and therefore it is essential to know what causes an imbalanced agni. Imbalances can happen overnight, but more often than not, it is a result of the habits that you may have formed. Many of these habits happen unconsciously, so it is important to become aware of your actions.

Perhaps one of the biggest mistakes you can make is overloading or burdening your agni. This happens especially when you overeat. Overeating slows down and weakens your digestive fire because your body is not able to efficiently digest food. Your stomach needs space to move around the foods, and your stomach muscles need to be able to contract and constrict as needed to be able to move the food along. For example, have you ever played the game called Fluffy Bunny? It's an American campfire game in which you stuff marshmallows into your mouth. As you go around the campfire, you keep adding one marshmallow to your mouth and try to say the words "Fluffy Bunny". Eventually your mouth is so stuffed that not only can you not speak anymore, but your jaw hurts and you can barely swallow or move anything around in your mouth. You end up most likely spitting out the marshmallows and never wanting to eat them again. This is what happens to your stomach if you overeat. When you fill your stomach entirely up with food, you feel so full that you may even end up feeling sick.

Other factors that weaken the digestive fire and can cause disease include eating before the previous meal has digested, eating too late at night, and not eating enough. In fact, Ayurveda would frown upon some of the new fad diets that revolve around fasting for extended periods of time. Eating breakfast should be just as important as your other main meals. Eating breakfast in the morning helps to kindle or light up the agni. It should not be the largest meal of the day, but it is essential to have because it really does break the fast. Skipping meals will weaken the digestive fire because without any fuel, the fire is not needed, and therefore it will also slow down your metabolism. Eating too late in the evening will keep your body from digesting the food well and will also disturb your sleep. Furthermore, if you eat before the previous meal has digested, this will overburden your digestion because it now has to begin to process the new food you are eating before it has fully worked through the first bits. Your body processes in the order that it comes through, but if something else is ingested before you fully digest the first bits, then your body will forget about the first bit and move onto the second bit. Ultimately, you may not be able to absorb all the nutrients that you have eaten.

Eating when you are feeling stressed, anxious, worried, or grieving, or during any emotional state, means your digestion will not be focused on processing what you are eating. Reflecting back to the role of the nervous system, if you are feeling any sort of emotional upset, your body is focused on fighting or running, and therefore it is not a good time to eat. Yes, there are exceptions to this, but in general it's best to eat only when you are emotionally settled. Stress causes all sorts of havoc, and eating when stressed may provide you with temporary comfort, but for your long-term health, it simply is not worth it.

Smoking, drinking, and the usage of illegal drugs is another factor that will upset your agni. In fact, all three of these are considered to be tamasic by quality. This means that rather than promoting balanced health, all three will do quite the opposite. Modern science fully backs this up. Those who smoke are fifteen to thirty times more likely to develop lung cancer and die from it than someone who does not smoke.[22] The use of drugs is also linked to mental health problems such as paranoia, depression, anxiety, low self-esteem, and more.[23] Furthermore, 20 per cent of all heavy drinkers go on to develop liver disease.[24] Therefore, it is important to avoid all three. Yes, red wine has some benefits that have been noted, but this is in small amounts. When it comes to making healthy choices, it is healthier to not include any alcohol, tobacco, or illegal drugs to keep your mind, body, and spirit healthy.

Within my clinical practice, I work with a lot of prediabetic and diabetic patients, particularly type 2 diabetic clients, and I often find that many of their blood sugar imbalances are a result of a weakened digestive fire. I can often see a clear connection between one of the causative factors and their health troubles. This is why diets do not work. I keep saying this because diets are not holistic, and there are so many factors to consider when it comes to your health. Without due consideration of routine, current eating habits, times that you eat, stress levels, sleep, and thorough analysis of your digestion, results cannot be achieved. If you interviewed every client I have ever had, they would all tell you that at their first meeting with me, I asked about their digestion and particularly their bowel movements. Healthy results can be achieved without any stress if you keep your digestion strong.

This may all sound complicated, but in the coming chapter, I am going to go through in more detail the action steps that you can take. I believe in educating and providing the foundation of knowledge. My clients will also tell you that I do not simply tell them what to do—I educate along the way so that they know why they are doing something. Knowledge is gold. Moving forward, I want you to keep in mind that you can easily adapt the Ayurvedic recommendations into any other plan. However, it is all about prioritising and making small changes one at a time. Start small and work your way up. Make a list and start with the things that appear to be the easiest for you. Then change things out one at a time. You do not have to make all the changes in one go. Like people say, slow and steady wins the race. Making changes is about nurturing your health and growing with it as needed. Be adaptable and open to change.

YOUR DIGESTIVE AND IMMUNE SYSTEMS ARE THE MOST IMPORTANT

By now, you have noticed the heavy emphasis on your digestion. The truth of the matter is that you must keep your digestive system strong and healthy. There is no other way around it, and this is true regardless of what your ultimate health goals are. Whether it's about losing weight, having thicker hair, balancing your blood sugar, lowering your cholesterol levels, or boosting energy levels, it all comes back down to your digestion. Take a moment and think about the following questions: How strong is your digestion? How well do you really feel after you eat? Food should not cause any discomfort whatsoever. Meals should always be pleasing to all your senses and provide nourishment.

This also means that no major food groups should be eliminated unless you are allergic or intolerant to it. Another exception is if you lack any particular enzymes that keep you from digesting a particular type of food. I cannot emphasise enough how important it is to not eliminate any particular food groups without the help of a qualified health or medical professional. For example, personal trainers should not give specific nutrition advice unless they have the qualifications to do so. Likewise, if you do any additional testing, know the efficacy before proceeding with it. I have had clients remove foods from their diets because they did a hair analysis to test for food allergies. These types of test, like the Vega test, are very temperamental and are not accurate at all.[25] You may as well randomly draw food names out of a hat, and those are the ones you are allergic too. There is no science behind those tests because they cannot test for the specific markers for food allergies or intolerances. If you do the test with two different specialists two days in a row, you are likely to get very different results. Invest in your health, but do not look for quick or unverifiable approaches.

Leaving out any major food groups without a proper reason and guidance can lead to severe nutritional deficiencies. With that said, having a balanced diet is important for having a healthy digestive system. This is where you want to follow the Ayurvedic principles of dietetics. These principles are the core values that should be upheld, and if you are looking for the place to start with regarding implementing more of Ayurveda in your day to day life, then this is where you want to begin. The principles sound simple but have a very powerful effect because they help keep the digestion strong, and that is nourishing for the mind, body, and spirit. How you eat is just as important as what you eat. You should always sit down to eat in a settled and quiet atmosphere with a settled mind. Light conversation is fine, but avoid any heated or passionate discussions. This also allows you to pay attention to your meal. With your attention on your meal, it becomes easier to recognise when you are full and satisfied, which helps prevent overeating.

My client Sherry first came to me for her chronic eczema. She had it as a child, and it got worse as she went onto adulthood. She had tried seeing all sorts of specialists, including a chiropractor, who had her eliminate foods based upon her hair analysis. Needless to say, that did not work. She then swapped to an osteopath, who referred her to me, and we did a proper blood test and discovered her food allergies and intolerances. As we worked together to eliminate those foods and ensure that her meals were nutritionally balanced, Sherry learned a lot about the principles of dietetics according to Ayurveda. She began to follow them and always sat quietly to eat her meals. However, at first her husband was reluctant to follow suit because he loved to watch television while eating. Eventually, he came around and has noticed that he feels better after he eats as long as he pays attention to the meal. He stopped getting heartburn because he soon realised that his heartburn was a result of him overeating. He was not paying attention to his meals, so he was not listening to his stomach.

When I work with children and their families, I also encourage parents and caregivers to leave their devices out of the kitchen. Meals are meant to be quiet and settled affairs. This way children learn to eat with their full attention on their meal, and early on they are able to recognise their hunger cues. For children, they should not be force-fed, so do not measure their meal quantities because that creates unhealthy food behaviours. It is best if children tell you when they are full. This is why I am a huge fan of baby-led weaning. Just like adults, children also need to learn their own portion sizes for themselves. With your full attention on meals, you will likely eat at a more natural pace that is not too fast or too slow.

Eat about three-quarters of your capacity. Place your two open hands together slightly curved upwards, and that is about the size of your stomach. Now, you don't want to fill that up completely. Remember the Fluffy Bunny example? Leave some room for digestion to take place. You can always eat again in a few hours, but wait until your previous meal has digested. On average, it is OK to eat every three to four hours. Lunch should be your main meal of the day, breakfast is a medium-sized meal, and dinner should be the lightest of all. Do not rush through your meals and snacks. Take the time to chew well because the digestive process begins in the mouth. The more your food breaks down in your mouth, the easier it is for your stomach to process it.

Be sure to include all the six tastes at every meal, but favour the tastes for your dosha. Regardless of which dosha you are attempting to pacify, avoid ice-cold beverages and foods because anything cold will completely weaken the digestive fire. In addition, it is best to favour cooked foods over raw foods. The exception is that those who are a strong pitta with a tikshna agni would do well with more raw foods because the stronger fire benefits from a greater challenge. The raw foods help balance and reduce the tikshna agni, thereby aiding in nutrient absorption. Those with a visham and especially a mand agni should avoid raw foods and unripe fruits as much as possible. Small amounts of raw foods are OK but should not be too often. Organic, fresh, and wholesome foods are nourishing for the digestion and immune system. These type of foods are also more nutritiously rich.

Eating at regular times throughout the day every day of the week is very beneficial. The body and especially the digestion system love regularity. By being regular with your meal and snacks times, this will prevent you from skipping any meals. Skipping meals can also cause blood sugar imbalances and can greatly affect your energy levels and your hormones. As you establish a regular eating pattern, this will also help kindle your digestive fire so it is always ready to digest when you sit down to eat. Once you eat, sit and relax for a few minutes. Allow the food to settle a bit before you get back up. This list is by no means exhaustive. These principles of dietetics are quite intuitive because they implement a level of mindful eating. Being aware of the choices you make and how your food choices make you feel will take you a long way.

When you begin to implement these principles, a good way to know whether or not this is working for you is to monitor your bowel movements. According to Ayurveda, you should have at least one bowel movement a day that is easy to pass and well formed. Ideally this should happen first thing every morning. It is best to start your day feeling clean and empty on the inside. Western medicine says that you have to have at least three bowel movements a week, and anything less than that is considered to be constipation.[26] Ayurveda has stricter guidelines. Therefore pay attention. Up to three bowel movements a day is considered normal in Ayurveda. However, when you begin to feel constipated or have too many other indigestion-related symptoms, such as acid reflux, heaviness after eating, metallic taste in your mouth, bloating, dry bowels, or straining during a bowel movement, then you may want to consider a detox. Here is a checklist of potential symptoms that may indicate the need for a detox.

- poor bowel habits (frequent constipation, diarrhoea, or both)
- frequent undigested foods in stools
- stools frequently smell and are excessively foul
- feeling better if you do not eat
- chronic indigestion after eating
- often do not sleep well and wake up tired
- frequently cold for no reason
- frequently feel tired, worn out, or depressed for no reason
- need to loosen belt or wear looser clothing after eating, even without overeating
- feeling bloated after meals
- frequent belching or passing of gas
- energy levels fluctuate throughout the day
- experiencing extreme food cravings
- loss of strength
- feeling heavy
- feeling lazy (capacity for work, but no enthusiasm)
- no taste for food
- mental and physical fatigue
- mental fog

If you have experienced at least two or more of the preceding symptoms on a regular basis, then that is a sign you may have ama, or undigested food, which is considered to be toxic in Ayurveda. "The place where Ama resides gives rise to pain and becomes the origin for many diseases, because the Doshas associated with Ama spread all over the body."[27] Keeping your digestion strong and balanced will help prevent the build-up of ama, but if you do have ama, you can clear it out.

A gentle home detox can often work out quite well. An Ayurvedic home detox does not require fasting or any harsh diet. Rather, it is a form of clean eating in its purest form. A gentle detox means eating wholesome foods, relying on foods that are commonly found in your local grocery store, and utilising your spice cabinet. When eliminating ma, you want to have a light diet, meaning you should favour cooked foods and avoid foods that may be difficult to digest. Soup is often ideal to have for lunch and dinner because they are wholesome and nutritious. One week is often plenty of time to reset your digestion. For this one week only, avoid gluten, dairy, nuts, eggs, meat, seafood, processed and packaged foods, coffee, and black tea. You can have vegetable and lentil-based soups for your main meals, porridge with fresh fruit for breakfast, and vegetable sticks, fruits, seeds, and dairy-free yogurt as snacks. The idea is to clean out your diet and give your digestion a break to allow it to heal itself while keeping yourself nourished.

Detoxing too often is not recommended. If you detox frequently—more than once every three months—then that could weaken your digestion and metabolism rather than heal it. Ayurvedic detoxes are best done at the change of seasons or when you begin to experience the symptoms of ama. A more gentle way to cleanse on a daily basis is to have hot water with lemon. Hot water is great for maintaining the digestive system, and lemon has a cleansing effect. Generally, one cup in the morning on an empty stomach is sufficient. However, those who are pitta should be careful because too much lemon can aggravate the dosha. In that case, plain hot water should work just as well.

Harsh cleanses such as detoxing by drinking only smoothies or using detox shakes is not recommended. Drastic changes to your diet can leave you feeling weakened and will negatively harm your digestive and immune systems. Juice cleanses can also leave you with nutritional deficiencies. Detox shakes often contain hidden ingredients and additives. Just because it is gluten-free or dairy-free does not make it healthy. Something that states it is sugar-free may not contain sugar, but is likely to contain sweeteners, whether artificial or real. Some also contain hidden ingredients such as bulking agents or "natural flavouring", and let's be honest—who actually knows what natural flavouring is?

When it comes to detoxing, always keep in mind that you do not have to go hungry; it should contain balanced and nourishing meals, and it should be as close to eating wholesome foods as possible. Detoxing is not a painful process, and if anything, it should make you feel better. Yes, some people initially get withdrawals from the sugar and caffeine, but aside from that, within a few days, you should be feeling so much better than when you started. Unless advised to do so by a health practitioner, home detoxes are not meant to last more than a week.

The purpose behind keeping your digestion strong and free from ama is to keep ojas strong and lively. Ojas is what keeps your immune system strong. Ayurveda tells us that there are eight drops of ojas found in the heart, as well as half an anjali (half the amount of your two hands put together) circulating throughout your body. There are factors that improve your levels of ojas, and then there are factors that diminish it or weaken ojas. Keeping your digestion strong certainly helps to promote healthy levels of ojas, but your actions and choices also play a role.

Ojas contains very positive energy by nature, and therefore any sort of negativity, especially negative emotions, will weaken ojas. Along with that, stress, rushing around, fasting, lack of sleep, injuries, and consuming alcohol or drugs weaken the presence of ojas. Stress levels are the lowest and health is the strongest when you are feeling happy within yourself. There is this great quote by Eleanor Roosevelt: "No one can make you feel inferior or superior without your permission." I love this quote because you can also interpret this as no one can make you feel happy or sad without your permission. Oftentimes people count on others or a situation to make them happy—for example, having this particular car or getting a promotion at work. But the reality is that none of those things are guaranteed happiness, especially beyond the point of when that particular event actually happens. Once it occurs and you do get that promotion, what happens next? Therefore, focus on making yourself happy right now in the present moment. The best way to do this is to spend at least ten minutes a day doing something for yourself that brings you joy.

Gratitude is another excellent practice that allows you to enjoy the present moment. Expressing gratitude allows you to appreciate what you have now. Then when you begin to appreciate the smaller things that do bring you joy, you realise that in this moment, you do not need anything else. One of my favourite quotes is by Eckhart Tolle, who says, "Realise deeply that the present moment is all you ever have."[28] Gratitude allows you to do just that and to experience the present moment. Every day, take at least one moment in which you take a deep breath and say thanks for what it is that you do have. One of my all-time favourite challenges that I completed a few years ago is the 100 Happy Days Challenge.[29] The concept is quite simple: all you have to do is find one moment a day that makes you happy and brings you joy for one hundred consecutive days. The entire process is transformational and is worth a go.

Bringing about joy and expressing gratitude will help keep your immune system strong and your stress levels down. With these practices, it costs no money, and you have nothing to lose and everything to gain. These are lifestyle choices that you can make to help yourself live a healthier life. In addition, you can eat food that directly helps boost your immune system. Surely we can all agree that the healthier we eat, the better we feel. The greater we feel, the better our immune system works. It is a chain reaction. The prevention model is quite simple in theory.

Good food —> stable energy levels —> healthy digestion —> good absorption of nutrients —> healthy immune system

As you know from the previous chapters, your specific choices make a big difference in how you feel. Having a balanced diet is essential and this means to have a balance of all major food groups. When it comes to your immunity, there are specific known foods that support it. These group of nutrients are known as antioxidants, and they are worth every bit of hype that is given to them. Aside from improving immune function, antioxidants are known to lower risks of infections and cancer, and they prevent tissue damage in the body that are caused by free radicals. Free radicals are cells that have been damaged and then harm healthy cells and DNA, which is what weakens the immune system and harms the body. Toxins and other chemicals that are found in the environment all cause oxidative damage to the cells. Asbestos, cigarettes, food preservatives, air pollution, drugs, pesticides, stress, and even intensive exercise cause free radicals to form.

That is correct: as wonderful as exercise is for your body, it does cause free radicals to form. Although exercise is great for managing stress and supporting the overall health of the body, there are downfalls. Intense exercise can cause oxidative stress, inflammation, and muscle fatigue.[30] Strength training especially causes extra formation of free radicals because it can tear and strain the tissues, muscles, and fibres within your body as you burn fat and attempt to create more muscle. It is a known fact that too much exercise can weaken your immunity. Because exercise creates free radicals, it is important that you focus on what you eat before and after you exercise to replenish your body. Eliminate the free radicals by eating foods that are high in antioxidants. Antioxidants will slow down, repair, and prevent oxidative damage to the tissues throughout the body.

Vitamin C is the most common nutrient that is associated with antioxidants. In addition, vitamin E, zinc, selenium, and carotenes are examples of nutrients that contain antioxidants. The list that follows is not exhaustive, but it includes examples of foods within each of the nutrients and the specific roles each of the nutrients play. Notice that there are plenty of options for each nutrient within your specific dosha food recommendations.

Vitamin C is commonly known for being an antioxidant and thus boosts your immune system, but it also helps with preventing free-radical damage, forms strong connective tissue, repairs wounds, improves gum health, and reduces bruising. Food sources include all berries, broccoli, guavas, kale, collard greens, capsicum peppers, watercress, cauliflower, persimmons, spinach, oranges, limes, and mangoes.

Vitamin E plays an essential role in supporting the brain, eyes, and cardiovascular health. Vitamin E also protects the skin. Food sources include wheat germ, sunflower seeds, almonds, sesame seeds, butter, spinach, oats, asparagus, salmon, and brown rice.

Zinc plays a role in protein and DNA synthesis, wound healing, bone structure, immune function, and skin oil gland function. Zinc is also important for healthy prostate tissue. Food sources include, oysters, red meat, poultry, ginger, pecans, Brazil nuts, eggs, whole wheat, rye, oats, peanuts, almonds, lima beans, and walnuts.

Selenium is an essential minerals that works alongside vitamin E. It helps to prevent cancer and heart disease and reduces heavy metal toxicity. Food sources include butter, wheat germ, Brazil nuts, scallops, barley, clams, oats, cow's milk, brown rice, molasses, and garlic.[31]

Carotenes are divided into two main categories, beta-carotene and alpha-carotene. Beta-carotene converts into vitamin A, and both are excellent sources of antioxidants because they both provide protection against cancer and cardiovascular disease. Food sources include carrots, sweet potatoes, squash, spinach, apricots, green peppers, mangoes, yams, apples, and peaches.[32]

I am not a huge fan of listing out antioxidant superfoods because superfoods are essentially nutritious food and can be open to interpretation. Yes, there are specific foods that are known to have cancer-fighting benefits, to give you an example, but when it comes to making healthy choices, it is not about selecting just one or two items off of that list in hopes that it will help offset any unhealthy choices you make. It is about following the eighty-twenty rule and eating foods that are overall healthy.

Therefore rather than promoting superfoods to my clients, I encourage them to eat a rainbow of colours. Eat a rainbow of colours each day, or at the very least throughout the week, and you will ensure that you get all your nutrients. You don't need to consume every single nutrient every day because our bodies use the nutrients as needed. As long as you eat a variety of colours throughout the week, you will get all the essential nutrients you need to protect your body and keep it strong.[33] Red is beetroots, apples, raspberries, radishes, and red peppers. Orange is sweet potato, oranges, tangerines, cantaloupe, and carrots. Yellow is lemons, onions, bananas, and yellow capsicum peppers. Green includes spinach, kale, cucumbers, avocados, kiwi, and asparagus. Blue and purple includes blueberries, aubergines, blackberries, raisins, and purple cabbage. The expert in eating a rainbow of colours is Dr Deanna Minich, who says, "Colour can heal your life." According to her expertise, red foods support adrenal health, orange foods help the reproductive system, yellow foods are excellent for the stomach and pancreas, green foods help the thymus and heart, and blue and purple foods support the brain and pituitary glands. In fact, she also adds a further two colours to get even more specific. The colour of aquamarine supports the thyroid gland and includes foods such as cucumber, elderberry, liquorice, and sea vegetables. White is the second added colour, which supports the pineal gland and cleansing; foods include coconut, garlic, white onions, parsnips, and sesame seeds.[34]

When you compare this list of foods high in antioxidants and the rainbow of colours to the forthcoming list of foods that promote ojas, you will see that there are quite a few similarities, which goes to show how strongly ojas is linked to antioxidants. Foods that are known to help increase the production of ojas are avocados, dates, figs, sweet potatoes, ghee, leafy greens, blanched almonds, other nuts (except peanuts), mung beans, pomegranates, sweet lassi (diluted yogurt drink with honey), rice, unheated raw honey, and boiled cow's milk.[35]

Aside from food, there are other ways to boost your immunity and levels of ojas. This comes back to routine and how you feel. Let's start with sleep. Getting your snooze in at night is highly recommended. There is so much truth to the old saying "Early to bed, early to rise, makes a person happy, healthy, and wise". Ayurveda has always encouraged that you should go to bed before 10.00 p.m. because between ten and two at night is when the body does most of its healing. Yes, that is pitta time of the night, which supports the healing process. In fact, modern science also says that the human growth hormone is predominantly released when the body is asleep, with the majority of the hormone being released before midnight, but it also takes about one hour from the time you fall asleep to begin releasing the hormone.[36] The human growth hormone is responsible for more than just growth; it also helps repair muscles, tissues, and cells, and most important, it helps regulate your metabolism. The earlier you go to bed, the more healing can occur.

Each dosha type has different requirements for sleep. Those with a vata imbalance will often have trouble falling asleep, and they need about seven to eight hours of sleep per night. Those with a pitta vikriti are generally light sleepers and can get by with less sleep; on average they need about six hours. Kapha people need a lot more sleep, often ranging from eight to ten hours of sleep. Remembering back to the dosha clock, it is still best to wake up before six in the morning, which means that kapha people would need to go to bed by eight in the evening to get ten hours of sleep. Know how much sleep your body needs and then adapt your routine so that your dosha can become balanced while getting in the hours of snooze needed for your body to repair itself from the day.

In order to stay on top of your immunity, you need to know how different foods and activities make you feel. This includes knowing what makes you happy. Happiness no doubt promotes immunity and boosts levels of ojas. On the days in which you feel stressed or saddened, you are naturally opening the door to weakening your immune system. Sure, sometimes you will feel sad, and you will need to experience the emotions and work through them, but on most days, it is important to know that happiness comes from within. Going back to the ten minutes a day that bring you joy, here is an experiential exercise that I would like you to try out. It is known as the Humour Collection. This can be in the form of a journal, box, or vision board. It needs to be tangible, so I encourage this to be something you physically put together rather than using technology.

Here are the instructions for the Humour Collection.

1. Collect items that make you laugh (e.g., comic strips, books, movies)
   A. If you only have a digital copy of the movie or book, write down the name of the book or movie on a piece of paper. I encourage you to decorate the paper, make it fancy, or print out a copy of the cover.
2. Collect items that make you smile or bring back happy memories (e.g., favourite holidays, pictures of family and friends, favourite places)
3. Put it all together in the form of a scrapbook or a large board, or into a box that is easily accessible.

As you can see, a Humour Collection is a compilation of items that make you happy. I have a notebook that I have created, but you are more than welcome to create a scrapbook, have a single board, or add the items to a box. Whatever method you use for your Humour Collection, I encourage that you allow space for it to grow and evolve as things change so that you can continue to add to it. The Humour Collection is something that you keep around that is easily accessible. On the days in which you are feeling down or sad for any reason, you simply refer to this to bring you a few moments of joy. In a way, this is also a reminder of all that you have that you are grateful for. Anything that can put a smile on your face is worth being a part of your Humour Collection.

Ultimately, we all want to feel happy and healthy. Laughter is scientifically shown to boost your immune system. Laughter engages the positive feeling which helps to fight stress and other illnesses. However negative thoughts set off a chain reaction in your body cause stress and thereby decreasing immunity. Laughing boost endorphins, which helps to reduce the feeling of pain, reduces stress levels, and improves your mood.[37] Do one thing every day that brings you joy and makes you smile. This will help keep your immune and digestive systems strong and nourished.

YOU MUST MANAGE STRESS LEVELS

When stress levels are high and you feel out of control, you may feel overwhelmed, get headaches, have fatigue, have trouble sleeping, have problems with concentration, experience short temper, overeat, undereat, experience food cravings for sugar or salt, have low energy along, and experience mood swings. On top of this, you may also experience eczema, psoriasis, and acne, and may have troubles with your digestion such as bloating, cramps, constipation, and diarrhoea. From this list, you can see that stress can lead to a variety of imbalances.

Let's be honest with each other. Stress is everywhere, and as much as I would love to say, "Let's prevent stress," this is not always realistically possible. Sometimes you take stress on yourself, but sometimes external situations give you stress. As I write this book, we are in middle of the Covid-19 pandemic, and I believe you will all agree with me that the pandemic has caused everyone a great deal of stress. This pandemic is out of our hands, and not one person has a control over it. That is why I feel that it is more important to manage stress than try to control it. Attempting to control stress will increase the feelings of it. It is essential to be able to release that which you have no control over. I truly believe that practicing mindfulness can reduce stress levels.

I introduced the concept of mindfulness in an earlier chapter, but I am mentioning it here again because we are now going to discuss how to incorporate mindfulness into your daily life. Part of mindfulness is letting go that which you cannot control and therefore living in the present moment. Living in the moment sounds very simple, but it is not. The first book I ever read about living in the moment was *The Power of Now* by Eckhart Tolle. He is one of the leaders in the movement of living in the here and now. Being present does not mean forgetting your responsibilities; it is about paying attention to the now. How many times have you walked down the same road and never noticed a tree on that road? How many times have you driven somewhere and not remembered exactly what happened or what you saw during your drive? We often do tasks on autopilot and go about mindlessly doing the things that we are so accustomed to doing without even thinking about them. Most often this happens when you are thinking about something else while performing another action. This is far from mindful living.

I was teaching a group yoga class when I lived in Bay Area, California. I was talking about living in the moment and not in our heads. I gave an example: "How often do you go back to check whether or not you locked your front door because you cannot remember?" I actually had a student leave because he started doubting whether or not he locked his front door. He never made that mistake again. It sounds so simple, but it is not. You doubt your actions simple because your full attention was not on the task at hand, and you were thinking about something else. Perhaps while locking your front door, you were thinking about the meeting you are going to, or you are worried about running late.

Focusing on the present can help reduce stress levels because usually the stress factor is out of your control. For example, if you have a half hour commute to work, you leave on time but unexpectedly hit traffic. This traffic means that you will be late for your meeting. If you start to get anxious and fidgety about it, nothing good will come of it. Inevitably, you feel stressed about it. But there is nothing you can do. Therefore, rather than thinking about being late for your meeting, focus on what can be done in the moment while you wait. Perhaps changing the radio station and listening to music will help you feel more at ease.

Living in the moment requires you to pay attention to yourself and to your environment. It means looking up and not looking down. Show interest and be curious about your surroundings. Put your phone away, and pick it up only if it is necessary. Very few—and I mean very few—people need to check their phones between parking their car and walking into their office. Nobody needs to check a phone when crossing the road. Stop multitasking. This in itself will help you live better in the moment. In fact, science says that our brains find it impossible to multitask. Rather, it is about how quickly our minds can go from one topic to another, moving back and forth.[38] This means that multitasking is actually quite taxing for the brain. When it all possible, do just one thing at a time.

There is a wonderful exercise I do with my clients when asking them to practice being more mindful and living in the moment. Whenever you find yourself getting lost into your thoughts or are having trouble focusing, you can do this short exercise using the five senses of sight, touch, sound, smell, and taste, which will bring you back into the moment. Here are the instructions for the exercise.

1. Depending where you are, your eyes can be opened or closed.
2. Take five deep breaths.
3. Starting with the sense of sight, identify at least two things that you may have not noticed recently within your range. If there is nothing new, take notice of any two objects that you can see.
4. Next, move to the sense of touch. Touch two different textures that are close by. Whether it's a brick wall during your walk, a flower in your garden, or the table at which you are sitting at, pick any two objects and notice how they feel.
5. Name two different sounds that you can here at the moment. Cars driving by, the washing machine, silence—it can be

anything. Yes, silence is a sound that is difficult to hear. What do you hear at the moment?

6. What can you smell? This one may be more challenging to pick two different smells, but give it a go. If you cannot pick two, even one smell will suffice.

7. What do you taste at the moment in your mouth? Can you still taste the morning coffee on your tongue? Or does your mouth taste dry? See if you can identify two tastes, but if not, pick at least one.

By noticing your senses and paying attention to how your senses are feeling, you are living in the moment. Tangibly, your senses can only identify what you are experiencing right now at this moment in time. In addition, another way to be present is by taking deep breaths. This is something that I always share with my yoga students in particular. When you take in a deep breath, it allows you to bring yourself back into the present moment, and each time you take a deep breath out, it is an opportunity to let go. Whenever you find yourself feeling any sort of stress, take a deep breath in and out and notice how you feel afterwards. Stressors may not go away, but you can certainly improve how you feel about them.

Meditation and relaxation techniques also help with managing stress. Meditation and relaxation are words that are thrown around these days, but what do they really mean? Meditation generally involves a specific technique that helps you to transform the mind. Oftentimes meditation will involve using a mantra or specific sound that will help you settle the mind while keeping your focus. Meditation techniques train the mind or induce a mode of consciousness that allows you to realise some benefit, or the mind can simply acknowledge its content without becoming identified with that content. It allows you to separate oneself from the ego and to experience higher states of consciousness. Meditation has a very specific end goal, and it is generally associated with liberating the soul or spirit and freeing yourself from the need of materialistic goods. With enough practice, meditation helps quiet the mind even when you are not meditating so that you can experience a constant state of contentment and feeling of peace.

Relaxation techniques are designed to free you from tension and anxiety. A relaxation technique is any method, process, procedure, or activity that helps you relax. It allows you to attain a state of increased calmness or reduce levels of pain, anxiety, stress, or anger. Colouring, listening to music, and yoga are just a few examples of relaxation. Meditation techniques can definitely help you relax, but not all relaxation techniques are considered to be meditations. I am not here to go into too much detail about the differences between the two, because ultimately I believe it does not matter what you choose as long as it achieves its purpose, in that it helps you feel better within yourself and be more of who you are.

Meditation and relaxation techniques do not have to be a religious or spiritual practice. Religion and spirituality are the same for many people, they are different for others, and perhaps they are nonexistent for some. Sure, you are welcome to associate religion or spirituality with the techniques you choose to practice, but you do not have to. My advice to all my students and clients is that meditation and relaxation techniques can mean something different to everyone, and therefore you have to choose one that works for you. There are numerous different techniques for both categories out there, but it is important to keep trying different ones until you find ones you enjoy. From my experience, the best practices are ones that you learn from a teacher or a guide. Meditation and relaxation techniques that you learn online can be good, but find one from which you can also learn and grow. Having a teacher or guide really does help because the more often you meditate or practice a form of relaxation, the more different experiences you will have. You will want someone there who can help you and be with you on your journey every step of the way.

The truth of the matter is that for a mindfulness, meditation, or relaxation technique to work and help you manage your stress, you must practice it with consistency. This is why you need to find a technique that you enjoy and that feels beneficial. If the practice feels like a chore, you will disengage from it and will not prioritise it into your daily routine. However, if the practice brings you joy, and you feel good for doing it, believe me when I say that you will end up prioritising it so that it becomes a part of your daily life. These techniques work, and there is plenty of science to back them up. Numerous research[39] studies show the benefits of meditation and relaxation, from improved health and sleep to better focus and greater productivity. Plus, through a regular practice of meditation or relaxation, you can help to balance all three doshas. A Zen proverb states, "You should sit in meditation for twenty minutes every day - unless you're too busy; then you should sit for an hour." Meditation makes you so much more productive that you will have hardly noticed you did not spend that time working.

Diet and lifestyle also play a significant role in managing stress. Being aware and mindful of how you are feeling will take you a long way. Meditation, relaxation, and mindfulness techniques teach you more about yourself. I keep coming back to this point because you want to be able to recognise how different situations, experiences, and foods make you feel so that you can be proactive about your health. Know what works for you and what does not, and when possible, choose to do the things that make you feel better and happier while balancing your responsibilities. Stress is everywhere, and we all have to face it, but learn which techniques help you to cope better.

When it comes to food, be able to identify what your comfort foods are and what you tend to reach for when you are under stress. Generally speaking, high-stress situations will often lead to cravings for foods such as carbohydrates, in particular breads and pasta, or foods that are high in sugar, such as cookies and cake. These may satisfy you short-term, but it will not help your stress levels in the long run. The truth is the cleaner you eat, the better you will feel. Remember antioxidants? These are also your friends under high-stress situations. Knowing your weaknesses allows you to also be better prepared. If your job is generally high stress, keep a stash of dried fruits and nuts so that you can eat those instead of a chocolate bar when you are feeling stressed. Dried fruit will also give you the sugar rush but without all the additives and additional refined sugars and sweeteners of a milk chocolate bar. The healthier you eat, the calmer you will feel. In addition, if you eat according to your dosha type, you will feel more balanced and therefore more in control over your thoughts and emotions.

Excess consumption of caffeine can make you feel more stressed than you are because caffeine increases the amount of cortisol and adrenaline released into your body. Many caffeinated drinks also cause a sugar and insulin spike, which makes you feel more on edge. Caffeine should be kept to a minimum, especially when you are stressed. However, having herbal teas instead could be beneficial. Chamomile tea, for example, is known to help you relax. Passionflower, green, and rose herbal teas can be very soothing. One to two cups of tea or coffee a day is fine, but anything more will aggravate the doshas and will not help reduce stress levels. Caffeine makes you feel better at first by giving you a boost of energy, but then it can lead to a crash and a feeling of weakness once the effects wear off.[40] If you drink more than two cups of caffeine a day, then slowly swap over those extra cups to decaf and eventually transition to herbal teas.

Exercise should be a key component of your lifestyle. Exercising the mind as well as the body should be a part of your daily routine. Physical exercise is known to help blow off steam and burn energy. Other benefits include improved strength and endurance, cardiovascular health, and immunity. Those who exercise at least thirty minutes a day, five days a week can better handle their stress than those who do not.[41] Exercise helps the body, calms the mind, and feeds the spirit. The time you spend exercising also allows you to often forget your challenges, and it is a wonderful practice in living in the moment. Take boxing for an example. It is a great form of physical and strength training that helps build resiliency. In the process of training, boxers learn to be in the moment to be ready to defend themselves when in the boxing ring.

This comes with practice. Exercising on a regular basis helps lighten the load in the mind so that you can focus on what is happening at this moment. Have you ever noticed that when you walk away from your problems, take a short break, and then return, all of a sudden your solution presents itself? It is all about giving your mind the break it deserves to refresh and gain a different perspective.

Knowing all these modalities of managing stress is great, but applying them is where it really counts. This is the time to reflect back, and I would like you to answer the following questions.

- What do you do at the moment to manage your stress?
- Is this working for you? Or do you feel that more needs to be done?
- Are you aware of how you are feeling? Do you engage in mindfulness/meditation/relaxation?
- How do you generally respond to stress and anxiety?

Once you have the answer to these questions, it all comes back to prioritising. If you feel that you do not engage in any mindfulness and are not managing your stress well, you must find ways to help yourself. Meditation or relaxation techniques are a great place to start. If you want to start small, there are numerous apps out there that help to calm you down and allow you to feel better. The downside of using apps is that you must make the time and keep yourself motivated. Initially it is difficult to get started, but once you have a routine down, then it is relatively easy to keep up with it. Another option is to have a meditation or relaxation buddy. This way, you can do it at the same time every day together; even if you live in different places, check in with each other afterwards, saying that you have done your daily practice.

Other great ways to manage your stress include getting outside. Go out for a walk or even sitting outside in your front yard or back garden can do wonders for your stress and mood. Fresh air is a great way to calm the nerves and feel more at ease. When possible, do your exercise outdoors. You get the double benefit of being outdoors and exercising. I have clients who will go for a walk with their umbrellas when it is raining, or they stand on their front porch just to breathe in some fresh air. Start with five minutes a day and work your way up. Incorporating your outdoors time into your daily routine is another approach that works. Consider walking to the high street if you are close enough rather than driving, or park your car farther away from the entrance. If you take online fitness classes and the weather is suitable, set yourself up outside to take the class. These are just some ways to get more fresh air.

In Ayurveda, prana is the breath or life force. It is what keeps you going. When you are worked up or panicking, how often does someone say to you, "Just take a deep breath"? We use this saying all the time, but we rarely stop to think about what these words actually mean. Taking deep breaths is very calming for the nerves. Here are a couple breathing exercises that you can try.

Deep breathing: This exercise is a slight variation of the Bhastrika, or Bellows Breath. Begin by sitting in a comfortable position. You can sit in a chair or sit cross-legged on the floor. Relax your hands onto your lap or legs, and relax your shoulders as you sit nice and tall. Close your eyes. Take a deep breath in through your nose, allowing your chest and stomach to expand. Hold your breath. Then deeply breathe out through your nose, allowing your chest and stomach to relax back in. You want your exhalations to be longer than your inhalations. To help with this, count your breath. Breathe in for five counts, hold your breath for five counts, and exhale for seven counts. If this feels fairly easy and breaths are not as deep, then breathe in for seven counts, hold your breath for seven counts, and exhale for ten counts. Do this deep-breathing exercise for five to ten minutes.

Pranayama: Officially knowns as Nadi Shodhana Pranayama, alternate nostril breathing is a great technique that is easy to do and can help you feel calm and settled. To do this breathing exercise, sit in a comfortable position, either on the floor on a chair with your back upright and your shoulders relaxed. Relax your left hand. Take your thumb and middle two fingers of your right hand and place them fingers on your nostrils. Your thumb should be placed on your right nostril, and your two middle fingers are on your left nostril. Your pointer finger should be pointing towards your third eye, in between your eyebrows. Begin by closing your left side of the nostrils and inhale deeply through the right side. Close both sides of the nostrils as you hold your breath for a few moments. Then open the left side of your nostrils as you exhale deeply. Then inhale through your left side, close both sides, and exhale through the right. Repeat. Do this breathing exercise for five to ten minutes.

Last but not least, your food choices will definitely affect how you feel. Follow your dosha pacifying diet and aim to eat balanced meals and snacks. Be sure to eat carbohydrates, protein, and healthy fats. Omega-3s in particular are excellent for reducing stress levels. If you do not eat fish, you can still get your healthy fats naturally by eating foods such as avocados, nuts, and seeds. When stress levels rise, so do your blood sugar and insulin levels. Therefore, protein consumption becomes even more important. Eating protein with your carbohydrates, even if its fruit or vegetables, this will help stabilise blood sugar levels. This is why food combinations such as apples and almond butter, carrots and hummus, and grapes and cottage cheese work so well together. They are all examples of carbohydrates combined with protein that will help stabilise your blood sugar levels, in turn helping you feel nourished yet calmer.

BEING HEALTHY IS ABOUT FINDING THE BALANCE OF REST AND ACTIVITY

The truth is that everyone needs to take a break and engage in self-care. People need time for themselves, but what does that really mean? What about when others depend on you personally or professionally? In one case, you are taking care of family, and in the other, you are nurturing your job. Either way, you are being asked to do more than you feel that you are capable of doing. Perhaps neither situation resonates with you personally, but at one point or another, you have felt that you were being stretched thin and did not have enough hours in a day. Students often feel this way, especially around exams time. At one point or another, everyone has been in a situation where one feels that one has too much to do and not enough time. Stress presents itself in all sorts of different ways, but when you feel that you are in desperate need of a time out, then that is a red light signal saying, Stop right now and take a break.

The key to balanced health is prevention, right? Ideally you want to take enough breaks along the way so that you do not get a red signal shoved into your face. Let's take the flu for an example. It starts with mild flu like symptoms such as a body ache and general feeling of being unwell. As the symptoms are mild, you decide to continue as per normal and go to work. Sure, you feel a bit rough, but it's nothing that you cannot plough through, right? The next day, you now have a new symptom of a headache, so you take some paracetamol and hope for the best. You cannot take time off from work because you have a deadline. There is no fever yet, so you decide to continue going to work and giving it your all. The next morning, you can barely wake up and have a high fever. Now you must stay home. By trying to plough through the initial signs, your symptoms only got worse, which now takes you off your feet for even longer. Imagine what would have happened had you taken a day off to rest, drink plenty of fluids, and have soup. It is likely is that you would have felt better much sooner. If you do not take breaks, your body will end up screaming at you until you do.

There is a reason why some mothers hide out in the bathroom for ten minutes at a time. There is a reason why many corporate executives block out their calendars for thirty minutes at a random time of the day. There is a reason why some people come home ten minutes later than expected from work. Their excuse is that they are carving out some time for themselves. I have a nutrition client who works full-time while raising two young children. Once every couple of weeks, she takes a morning off from work and spends that time getting her nails done, going for a haircut, getting a massage, reading a book, or doing anything else that she feels like getting done. She has never had to explain her time off because she does plan them, but this is how she manages to get a few hours to herself to do whatever she wants to do.

Sometimes you have to get creative in how you incorporate it, but everyone needs a bit of a time out, a break from life, and a break from reality. Here is how to do that. First of all, start by switching off your devices so that you can ensure you are not disturbed. If you are having trouble turning your phone off because you are afraid of getting a call from your kids or an elderly parent you take care of, a great way around this is to put your phone on Do Not Disturb mode and selecting the option to allow calls from your favourite lists. Most phones have this feature. The idea here is that you want to switch off and disconnect without having to worry. Do this for about five minutes to start with. If you are planner, schedule in the time into your calendar. Block off that time every day; it can be at different times, but plan for at least five minutes a day. Then choose an activity that you enjoy. For example, for five minutes you will read a magazine while soaking your feet in a foot bath. Or you will do five minutes of a breathing exercise. It is important to start with five minutes and gradually raise it to thirty minutes that can be done anytime of the day. I have clients who meditate on their train journey into work. I have clients who read a book while their food is being baked in the oven. In order to make time for yourself, you may have to get creative and perhaps even stay firm. Communicate with your partner that your self-care time is nonnegotiable. Then commit to yourself that you will do this. No one can force you to take care of yourself. This is on you, so choose to make yourself a priority and stick with it. You can even do something different every day, but do it.

Earlier in the book, I shared with you about how overuse, underuse, and misuse of time, senses, and actions are the causative factors for illnesses. It is important to stay active while also taking breaks. There is such a thing as exercising too much. Too much exercise will fatigue the body, and you need to allow time for rest and recovery. I had a client we'll call Janet. She was really into fitness and training and therefore was very active. When I met her, she was seeing her personal trainer four times a week, and on top of that she was taking martial arts classes three times a week because she was working her way up to becoming a black belt. She ran a 5K twice a week and had nearly twenty thousand steps a day. Janet was also drinking large amounts of protein shakes. Her goal was to tone up and get fit. She started her journey strong and well, but as the weeks went on, she felt tired all the time and started getting adult acne. Upon my initial intake for Janet, I found out that she developed digestive issues, including constipation and heartburn.

It is clear that Janet loves her physical activities and enjoys everything that she does. In fact, she considers her daily exercise her "me time". Her chiropractor had referred her to me for her nutrition, and I gave her two main pieces of advice. She needed to incorporate some rest time, and she needed to eat more real food while reducing her use of protein shakes. I explained to her that she needed more healthy food, including plenty of fruits, vegetables, and real-food sources of protein. I also explained to her why she needed to have a diet high in antioxidants. As we worked together, we focused on healing her digestive issues, and Janet began to feel more energetic. She also eventually swapped her 5K runs for my yoga classes and included more rest days into her lifestyle.

In many ways, yoga is the perfect form of exercise that incorporates both rest and activity. A classical or hatha yoga class will often begin with a short meditation or relaxation exercise, which will go into breathing exercises. Then there will be a physical practice of yoga asanas or postures, and finally the class ends with savasana, which is a form of relaxation while lying flat on your back. Yoga encourages movement and taking breaks in between certain postures. There are plenty of relaxation poses in yoga that students can take part in at any time. The rest times in yoga or outside the times of other exercises is crucial because that is the time your body gets to heal itself. Sure, you can keep going and going, but remember that everyone needs a break. Even body builders have days off from training.

During the rest days, it is still important to stay active, but not as vigorously. There are other ways to stay active without necessarily overdoing the exercise. This includes ensuring that you stand up and move every hour. This is especially important if your job or daily routine is quite sedentary. You can even set up a reminder on your computer or phone that nudges you to take a break every hour. The five-minute break will double the time of productivity to your day. Walking is very helpful. The average recommendation is to take ten thousand steps per day, which is a good goal for most people. If you have a pedometer or a fitness tracker, you can keep track of your steps. Going for a leisurely walk can also be beneficial. Not all forms of exercise need to be intense. On your days of rest, stay active, but be slightly more relaxed about it.

Walking has its benefits. Walking is known to help maintain a healthy weight, strengthen the bones and muscles, improve mood, help with balance and coordination, and prevent heart disease, high blood pressure, and type 2 diabetes.[42] Walking is also great for digestion and relaxation. Especially if you go for a walk outside, it helps you to relax and feel rejuvenated. You can even do this with a friend. Going out for a coffee or a meal with friends is very common, but you can sometimes make these meet-ups more productive by making it an active one. If you are meeting a friend for a coffee, instead of sitting at a coffee shop, why not go for a walk instead? You can still buy your coffee, but drink and walk at the same time. This means that you are staying physically active while meeting a friend.

Being active and resting are essential for achieving balanced health. The way we use our time, how we engage our senses, and the actions we take all affect our health. For example, instead of going to bed on time on a weekday night, if you choose to stay up late to binge-watch your new favourite television show, you are now overusing and misusing your time, senses, and actions. Instead you should be sleeping and getting the rest that you need.

Sleep is the time when the body repairs itself. Mark Black once said, "Sometimes the most productive thing one can do is to relax." A variation of the quote that is also used just as frequently is, "Sometimes the most productive thing one can do is to sleep." Rest time, and particularly sleep, is of the utmost importance. Although it sounds easier to push sleep aside, it does have adverse effects on your health. Proper sleep brings about happiness, nourishment, strength, and life. Sleep should never take a back seat because we all know what it feels like when we do not get a full night's sleep. With a lack of sleep, you feel tired and less productive. You also decrease your body's ability to work efficiently, and you compromise your immune system. Therefore, make sleep a priority and do not push it aside.

If you suffer from insomnia, or you have trouble falling asleep or staying asleep, it is important to find the root cause of your sleep challenges. At this point, you also want to look at your daily routine, including exercise. Take an even closer look at what you are eating and drinking. I have a client who cannot fall asleep, and it had been like that for years. Once he started exercising, all his sleep challenges disappeared. We were able to make a clear connection that as long as he exercised three to four times a week, he was able to sleep just fine. His body needs the exercise to burn the excess energy he has and clear his mind so that he can sleep.

Other great ways to improve sleep are to avoid any caffeine after lunchtime; for those who are incredibly sensitive to caffeine, this means avoiding chocolate and green tea as well. Eating lighter dinners and allowing two to three hours to digest before sleeping is also helpful. Avoiding any screen time up to one hour before bed can improve sleep. I also have clients who drink less water after about six in the evening, which means that they are not having to use the toilet as much at night. Drinking vata tea, chamomile tea, and other herbal teas can help with sleep quality. There are sleep-time guided meditations that can be done. I have one client who listens to baby lullabies before going to bed. You can try any of these, and so much more, to help improve your sleep. If you are having trouble sleeping, it is best to troubleshoot and help yourself sooner rather than later.

You will always have time for something that is important to you. Therefore, be honest: How do you spend your time? Time management is something that I feel everyone should be well versed in. There are only so many hours in a day, and more often than not, most people feel that there is not enough time in a day to get everything done. You may find it helpful to write down and keep track of your entire day to see how you spend your time. This is useful in knowing which areas you can reorganise and where you have pockets of extra time. Many people find that waking up earlier is a good way to give themselves extra time, and that is when they get their "me time". My dad was always an early riser. He used to get up at 5.30 a.m. every day, even on the weekends and when he did not have to be at work. As a teenager, I once asked him, "Why do you get up so early?" He responded, "It's the quietest part of my day." I did not fully understand that until I started doing that in my late twenties, and I realised just how peaceful, relaxing, and productive those early morning hours are.

Reorganise your time if you need to, but ensure you schedule in that time for yourself. I know that by fine-tuning your levels of rest and activity, you will have more energy, and your stress levels will drop. Create a routine and be consistent. In an ideal world, you will have your exercise and rest times at the exact same times every day. However, that may not always be possible. Therefore, to be realistic, prioritise your sleep times to be consistent so that it helps with establishing your circadian rhythms, which will definitely help if you have sleep troubles. Exercise may not be at the same time every day, but if you aim to exercise the same days of the week, that is a good place to start. For example, exercise every Monday evening, Wednesday afternoon, and Friday morning. This may not be a consistent time daily, but it is consistency weekly. Consistency does not have to be the exact same thing every single day of the week, but you do need structure. Within that structure, be sure to schedule in rest and activity.

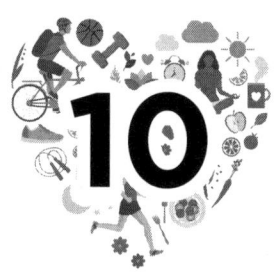

YOU CAN HAVE A LIFESTYLE THAT MAKES YOU FEEL YOUR BEST

I know from my years of experience that lifestyle changes do work, and to some extent, lifestyle is a greater influence than your dietary intake. Your lifestyle will also influence the type of food choices you make. The way you live your life is also influenced by your external environment, such as those you reside with or work with, where you go to work, and how you spend your personal time. All these factors need due consideration when making changes. I always ask my clients whom they live with and how supportive those people are with the changes that they made need to make. I also ask my clients if their family members would be willing to adapt any dietary changes as a way to support them but also to make life easier, in that only one dish needs to be prepared for everybody rather than everyone eating something different.

In order to feel better within your mind, body, and spirit, you must be open to making changes. Realise that this journey to better health will constantly change. The plan you create for yourself today may be different than the plan you have for yourself next month. As your circumstances change, you may find that you need to make other changes. As you establish new habits, you may want to build upon that and add new habits to your daily routine. Regardless of where you start your journey, be open to change and modifying along the way. Along with being flexible about the changes you make, be realistic. Know where you are starting. If your goal is to lose weight, write down your current weight, write down your goal weight, and then calculate how much weight you want to lose. Take that number and add four. This is how many weeks it will take you to lose the weight, on average. If you took your weight in pounds, then divide the amount by two. You want to aim to lose no more than one kilogramme or two pounds per week. For example, if you want to lose fifteen kilogrammes, then it will take at the very least nineteen weeks to lose the weight. On your weight-loss journey, you will face obstacles and weeks where the weight loss will plateau; this is your body signalling you that you need to change things up. Your diet or exercise regimen may need updating. Do not expect a straight decline in weight; this rarely happens.

Weight loss is not about dieting. It is about finding yourself while you make dietary and lifestyle changes. I truly believe that when you decide to lose weight, it is about the journey of discovering the healthier you, and the weight that drops off is an added physical bonus. If you want to lose weight, be considerate of your age, starting weight, dosha, and any other health challenges that you may have. Also be mindful of the fact that in addition to healthy eating, your exercises should include strength, cardio, endurance, and flexibility. You need all four parts for a holistic fitness plan.

Perhaps one of your goals may be to eat less sugar or snack less frequently. For either of these goals, recognise why you engage in this behaviour. Why is it that you like sweet foods? Why is it that you are always snacking? Then you must create a plan as to how will you stop. And why do you want to stop? Without having a strong enough why, chances are that you will not be able to stop. There are numerous ways out there to help reduce your intake of sugar and snacks, but you must find a way that works for you. One thing that does work for majority is having a support system. Regardless of what change you want to make, there are two things you must have in place. Be able to answer the following questions: Why you want to make this change? Who is in your support system?

Be patient with the goals that you set yourself. To achieve lasting results, it takes time and perseverance. Be realistic about your goals. Another factor to consider is your health history. How long have you had this problem? If you have been suffering from irritable bowel syndrome for five years, do not expect the problem to go away in five days. It takes time to repair and heal. Your medical history is just as important as how you are feeling today. List out all the aspects of your health and habits that you do not like. There is no limit to how long your list is, but write down everything that you would like to change. Be detailed as possible so you know where you are starting from. Once you have your list, pick and choose your priorities. Circle or star your top five priorities or health goals. Then from here, pick and choose your top two or three priorities. If you have twelve things on your list that you want to change about yourself, you cannot do all that all at the same time. This is why you have to prioritise. What is the most important change for you to make? What is it that you value the most? This is your starting point.

I have always believed that it is the smaller steps that make the biggest difference. I tell my yoga students that there is no point in being able to do a fancy impressive asana or pose if you cannot do the steps in between and hold the pose along the way. The journey to the pose is where the growth happens. Throughout this book, I have not laid out a perfect diet plan or a lifestyle, but I have given lots of possible options for you. In the next chapter, I will show you my formula for creating your ideal plan at home, but before you do that, you need to know why you are making the changes that you are.

As a part of these smaller steps, create your own ideal daily routine. You know what the ideal daily routine consists of according to Ayurveda, but what works for you? Write it down. List everything that you want to include in your daily or weekly routine. No detail is too small, so write it all down. Then from here, prioritise. Circle or star your top five things you want to include in your routine and then highlight the top one or two items. Personally, I feel that you should set regular wake and sleep times as a starting point because this will become your baseline. However, this is easier said than done for some, so if this is not a priority for you, then do not worry about it. Eventually, though, you should consider this, especially if you have trouble sleeping.

Other factors you may wish to consider adding to your daily routine are mealtimes. Having the same meal times daily, including weekends, is great for digestion and helps balance all three doshas. Regular mealtimes also ensure that you plan ahead and are making the time to eat well. Consistency with your breakfast, lunch, and dinner times may require scheduling as well as self-discipline. I have a client who had a severe vata imbalance when we first met. One of the factors that really helped her balance her vata was eating at the same times every day, including weekends. Years later, she still follows a vata pacifying regimen because her tendency is that vata can become easily imbalanced. She says that the only things she can really control in her day are her sleep and wake times, along with mealtimes. That gives her the basic foundation for all her other healthy habits. Eating at the same times daily will help balance digestion and metabolism so that you can have a sama agni. Of course, eating according to your dosha type will also help with this.

Staying hydrated is another key consideration. The average recommendation is two litres of water a day, which is roughly sixty-four ounces. For a more precise amount, take your weight in pounds and divide by two; this is about how many ounces of water you should drink per day. This formula does not consider exercise, so if you are working out, you will want to drink more water. Considering your body is meant to be about 60 per cent water, staying hydrated is important to keep your kidneys functioning optimally, and it also helps with nutrient absorption. Being well hydrated also helps with having regular and well-formed bowel movements, as well as keeping your energy levels up. Caffeinated beverages, along with juices and squashes, do not count towards your water intake. In fact, if you are going to have any of those, I recommend having a glass of water before and after to ensure that you stay hydrated.

The other activities that you may want to consider being a part of your ideal daily routine are exercise, self-care time, and breaks. Remember that we all need a balance of rest and activity. Exercise is key, but so is downtime, so try to include both if you can. Otherwise, prioritise. Which is needed more? If you are on your feet all day, then maybe rest is more important than exercise. Or if you have a desk job, then maybe you need to consider exercising rather than resting. Be mindful of how your day is and then pick which one to consider. Either could be a part of your self-care. However, self-care also needs to be something that you truly enjoy. If you feel that rest is more important, be specific as to how you are resting. You could consider using art therapy as your form of self-care as well as your resting time. Art therapy comes in so many forms these days, ranging from a colouring app that you can download to painting by numbers. If you want to keep it simple, there are plenty of colouring book options that are designed for adults. This may be your chance to find your inner artist.

Exercise is ideally meant be at least thirty minutes daily or one hour every other day. It should get your heart rate up and include both cardio and strength exercises. Again, let's be realistic. Is this possible? If not, really ask yourself how much time you can commit. Even if it's five minutes daily, allocate that time for your physical health, which also provides benefits to your mental health. My approach has always been that five minutes is better than not doing anything. Start small and work your way up. Smaller goals are more achievable with lasting results than large goals that you cannot keep up with.

As a part of your lifestyle and routine, you also need to consider your nutrition and what you are eating. I do not like using the word *diet* because there are too many negative associations with it, even though diet is really meant to be more of a holistic word that simply refers to what you eat. There are lots of considerations to take in terms of eating healthy. It starts with finding the right balance. Try to maintain that balance of eighty-twenty I mentioned earlier. This means that you eat healthy 80 per cent of the time, and the remainder 20 per cent of the time, you allow yourself to deviate from the plan. The idea is not to limit or fully restrict yourself in terms of what you eat. Even within your vata, pitta, or kapha pacifying diets, follow the eighty-twenty rule. Keep in the mind the only foods you should refrain from eating are the ones that have been identified by a health professional that you are allergic or intolerant to. In other words, aim to have a positive association with food and know that food ultimately should make you feel good. If food does not sit well with you, seek help from a qualified nutritionist.

Remember that diets do not work, but making dietary and lifestyle changes does work. Set a goal to eat healthy, eat clean, and eat balanced meals. Aim to eat a variety of foods that are nourishing. You can eat anything you want as long as you have everything in moderation and follow the basic principles of dietetics. This will allow your digestion to stay strong. That is the secret key to eating anything. Have the digestive fire strong enough yet balanced to allow yourself to truly enjoy food.

As you work through and create your ideal daily routine, be sure to factor in sleep at some point. Many of you may feel that you can get by with less sleep, but being healthy is not about getting by—it is about feeling your best. Take the time to do some inner reflection and be completely honest with yourself. How much sleep do you really need? You can use your dosha as a starting point if you need some guidance. Part of sleep and bedtime is having a specific winding down, or what I like to call a prebedtime routine. This is what you do before you get into bed. This is the time to relax, switch off your devices (including the television), perhaps take a bath, do some reading (preferably using a physical book), colour, listen to relaxing music, engage in light conversation, or do simple bedtime stretches. The possibilities are endless. Studies show that screen time is not helpful for sleep, so if you have trouble sleeping or are always wake up feeling tired, consider changing what you do about one hour before you get into bed. Then your actual bedtime routine is what you do once you are in bed. Do you read some more? Do you do some breathing exercises or meditation? Or do you literally lie down straight away and go to sleep? Some people need some additional time in bed before going to sleep, and others can fall asleep immediately. Have a think and write down all the things you would love to have as a part of your prebedtime and bedtime routine. Then prioritise from the list you create.

BEING HEALTHY IS SIMPLER THAN YOU THINK

In the previous chapter, I gave you plenty of options as to where to begin, all of which are equally important. You may already do some of it, or perhaps you do none of it. The list may appear daunting, but remember that being healthy is simpler than you think. Being healthy and feeling healthy should not feel like a chore. Ultimately you must follow an approach that makes you happy and excited. The bottom line is that if you aren't happy, then no matter what you do, it will not work. That is why I ask you to prioritise and start with the changes that are most important to you. The changes you want to make have to mean something to you. One of the reasons you picked up this book is because whatever you have been doing until now has not been working for you. You are looking for something new. The unique part of my approach is that you get to create your ultimate plan. Many self-help books these days talk about creating your ultimate life and using the law of attraction. In many ways, I am asking you to do the same, except we are keeping the focus to your health and overall well-being. I am asking you to create the lifestyle that you would like to have, but you should also stay within your means. Then of course, make changes along the way as life is always changing.

Everything you do should inspire bliss. All actions should make you happy and therefore will nourish your spirit. One of the ultimate goals in life is to be happy and you can only really find true happiness when you feel that you are taking your life in the direction you want to go in. I have had cancer patients feel their absolute worse during the peak of their chemotherapy treatments, but what would make them happy is the routine that they would create for themselves—their self-care routine they would be able to do regardless of whether they were at home or at the hospital. Their self-care routine gave them hope and allowed them to feel in control, even if it is for that short time of the day. The choices you make should allow you to begin feeling better within yourself, and as long as that initial excitement is there, plenty more can come from it.

As you continue on this journey of simplifying healthy living, you must not believe everything you read. There is a lot of conflicting information out there. Science is constantly changing, and we are all learning new things every day. However, when it comes to your health, it is important that you trust only reliable sources. Believe it or not, social media is not the place to turn to for reliable information, and neither is any search engine. Yes, I am sure you have searched for your symptoms before, and you will continue to do so, but it is important to not make an assessment based upon what you have read or even heard. It is also worthy to note that you should trust yourself and listen to your intuition. If the advice does not sit well with you, get a second opinion.

I was at a social gathering when my son was about three months old. I met another mum, and we started talking about children because her son was a year older than mine. We were talking about night feeds, and she told me to wean my son at the age of four months so that he would sleep better, because that was what she did for her son. Although she meant well, there are two key points to note here. First, the advice she gave is potentially harmful for the long-term health for most babies. Second, she did not even know that she was speaking to a qualified nutritionist. I did end up telling her that I would not be doing that and laid out my reasons for why babies should not be weaned early unless mothers are told to do so by a qualified professional. She was taken aback, and all I can say is that I hope that she still is not giving out the same advice.

As a member of quite a few online social groups and networking communities, I see far too many people asking for advice on various groups. A majority of the time, people really do mean well, but their experiences are not always helpful. I understand that many times people turn to social media or social forums to get advice and help because they feel lost or stuck, but ultimately you should trust only reputable sources. Instead, ask for connections to qualified professionals. When choosing a path, keep it simple. Being healthy really does not have to be complicated. If you hear an approach that is a quick fix or too complex, question it. If you are being sold a large amount of products or supplements, ask yourself, "Is this really necessary?" Ask yourself how real the information that you are getting it. Can you verify it? Can the person recommending this to you send you verifiable information through a reputable source? I have a client who does just that. Anytime we speak about a recommendation I have for him or any new piece of information I share, he searches through reputable academic or scientific journals to see if he could verify the information from other sources.

Sometimes people try to do things themselves and find their own cures online. Yes, sometimes this works, but many times it does not. This is when you want to reach out and find a professional to help support you. There is a saying: "Even therapists have therapists." Do not feel that you have to go about finding balanced health on your own. This book will definitely give you the guidance to help you, but if you need even more help, reach out. Avoid making decisions based upon peer pressure or upon the latest trend. Trends will always come and go. I have always said the best trend would be if healthy living was simplified and if living a balanced lifestyle became popular. Diets do not work, and exercise alone does not work either. You really do need a little bit of everything ranging from healthy eating to exercise, rest, and self-care. Everything you do for yourself should be about nourishing the mind, body, and spirit. Be committed to the choices that you are making. Clients I have with the greatest success are the ones who are committed and all-in to begin with.

I have a series of health questionnaires that I send out to all my nutrition clients before working with them. In a way, this is a test for me to see how committed they are. When I initially started my nutrition practice, I would meet with clients regardless of whether or not they filled out the forms. The ones who did not fill them out were least committed to their health. They simply liked the idea of meeting with a nutritionist, but they seldom implemented any changes. Over the years, I learned from those experiences. Now, if a client does not complete those forms, I will not meet with the person. I keep saying this because that is how important it is: You must be committed to making the changes. This is your life, your health, and your choice. How you do it and why you choose to make healthy changes is up to you to decide.

Following this chapter, you will see a guided worksheet for you to complete. Using this book as a reference and implementing what you have learned, you will create your own plan based upon my guidance. This is the formula I often use with my clients to ensure that their goals are met.

Having a balanced intake of food and a perfect daily routine in an ideal world will result in you feeling your best, but the truth is that none of us live in a perfect world. As discussed earlier, stress is always there. It's a matter of how you cope with it. Some parts of your life may be out of your hands, but within your means, do the best you can. Do not try to make all the changes in one go. Humans are often resistant to too much change by nature, so be gentle. Share your journey with a friend, journal about your experiences, or share on social media. Part of my clients' successes are the fact that I have them keep daily food journals or hold them accountable for their choices. My clients know that they will be speaking to me, so that keeps them motivated. However, once you begin to notice the positive changes in how you feel, you will be able to keep yourself accountable. This is why documenting your journey in some way will show you how far you have come.

In addition, remain positive and surround yourself with people who uplift you. Believe in yourself, and others will believe in you too. Be true to who you are, where your journey has brought you to, and where you are going. Recognising and accepting your past helps you to build a healthier and happier future. Being a healthier version is all about you and nobody else. It may sound selfish, but it is far from that. You cannot give from an empty cup, so I cannot emphasise it enough about how important your choices are. Every choice you make, including even the outfit you pick for the day, influences how you feel. Therefore, choose that which makes you feel your best and empowers you. Ultimately, the healthier you feel within your mind, body, and spirit, the more you will feel energetic and empowered, and the more you will feel that you can do anything you set your mind to do.

As you continue on this journey to achieving balanced health, own the changes that you want to make. You do not have to justify these changes to anyone but yourself. Stand up for the plan that you are about to make. Own it and be proud that you have chosen to take your health and place it in your own hands. Make informed choices and trust the process. There is no such thing as a quick fix, so be patient. Long-term, lasting results take time. Start with your dosha and the advice that Ayurveda lays out. Pick and choose from these things. The four key areas are nutrition, activity, sleep, and self-care. Everything falls into at least one of these categories, and everything Ayurveda has to offer nourishes the mind, body, and spirit. No one can choose to live a healthy life for you—this is up to you to decide. Most important, have fun on this journey towards healthier living. The trip should be just as much fun as reaching the destination, because once you reach your destination, you have more things to do. This is why the lists you have made and the worksheet you are about to use will come very useful.

Healthy living is not an all-or-nothing approach, and a one-size-fits-all model does not work. That is why you need to create a plan for yourself that resembles you and prioritises your needs. If you start with one or two goals that are most important to you, then you can continue to grow and adapt from there. You do have a choice; it may not always be the most ideal of choices, but you always have a choice. Choose healthy whenever possible. Choose to care for yourself, and choose to put your own needs first when possible. The better you take care of yourself, the better you can take care of others. Be mindful of your choices and learn about how your choices make you feel. By making your own choices towards healthier living, you are empowering your own well-being.

I wish you all the greatest success in achieving and maintaining balanced health in a simplified way. Always remember that being healthy is simpler than you think, and health comes down to the choices that you make. Keep it clean, keep it fresh, keep it wholesome, choose yourself, and prioritise your health now and forever. I now recommend that you go on to fill in the "Creating Your Ideal Wellness Plan" on the next page.

CREATING YOUR IDEAL WELLNESS PLAN

In this section, please be as honest with yourself as possible. I have left you plenty of space to write your answers within the book. However, if you need more space, please use another sheet of paper.

What are your top five health concerns?
1.
2.
3.
4.
5.

What are your top five health goals?
1.
2.
3.
4.
5.

Do you have any health habits that you would like to change?
1.
2.
3.
4.
5.

What activity do you do, and what do you eat, when you are feeling:
- Bored?
- Happy?
- Angry?
- Lonely?
- Tired?
- Depressed?
- Celebrating?
- Hungry?

What were your dosha assessment results?

What are your priorities? Check all that apply, or write in your own.
- ○ Improve dietary/nutrition
- ○ Dosha balancing
- ○ Lose weight
- ○ Set a wake time
- ○ Regular bedtime
- ○ Eat breakfast at the same time every day
- ○ Eat lunch at the same time every day
- ○ Eat dinner at the same time every day
- ○ Create a morning routine
- ○ Boost water intake
- ○ Take regular breaks
- ○ Exercise more often
- ○ Engage in self-care
- ○ Eat more dosha balancing meals
- ○ Eat more protein, carbohydrates, or healthy fats
- ○ Have a bedtime or prebedtime routine
- ○ Quit smoking
- ○ Limit or reduce alcohol intake
- ○ Take at least ten thousand steps per day

- Do daily abhyanga
- Have a meditation practice
- Have a relaxation practicing
- Engage in mindfulness
- _____
- _____
- _____
- _____
- _____

What do you enjoy doing? What do you like to do? If you had an extra hour, how would you spend it?

Choose five items from the list of priorities.
1.
2.
3.
4.
5.

From the list above, pick up to two items to focus on.
1.
2.

How will you implement these two items? How much time will you dedicate for yourself?

This is your plan. If you have a support system, share it with people. If you want to keep it private, that is fine too. Be sure to schedule your plan if you have to, but make the plan as solid as possible. Schedule it in and prioritise you. Your self-care is not optional—it is a priority. These are the choices that you are making to improve your health and well-being, which starts right now.

ACKNOWLEDGEMENTS

Firstly, I would like to thank my parents, Vijay and Jyoti Solanki, without whom I would not have the knowledge or experience to write this book. From early in my childhood, I remember them saying to my brother and me that we should not eat sugary cereals or foods with added food colouring because they are not healthy. They also use many Ayurvedic and herbal home remedies, which I still remember. They have always supported me and helped me get through my undergraduate and graduate studies. I will always be thankful for all that they have done for me, and they helped me become the person I am today. They are the ones who inspired me to choose the path of alternative and complementary approaches to health care as my career.

I would like to thank all my professors during my undergraduate years, but in particular Dr Paul Morehead and Liis Mattik, who have taught me everything that I know about Ayurveda. They helped me build the foundation of knowledge from which my clinical experience arises.

Thank you to my yoga teacher, Shashi Pottathil, for helping to heal my mom but also for teaching me yoga and the true meaning and practice of it. He comes from a family of yoga lineage, so learning from him is as close to the purity of teaching as I can get. I still remember and pass down the knowledge that he taught me.

Thank you to my teachers in graduate school, but in particular Linda Clark and Paula Svloboda, who taught me everything about health education and nutrition. They allowed me to also integrate nutrition and Ayurveda with many of my assignments. This supportive learning helped me build my business and clinical practice, Illuminated Health.

I would also like to thank all my nutrition clients, yoga students, workshop attendees, and course students, without whom I would not be as successful as I am today. Thank you for trusting me with your health and well-being. A big thank-you to those who have also allowed me to share their stories. I have changed their names and other identifying details to protect their privacy.

In order to turn this book from an idea to actual tangible work, I would like to thank Mindy Gibbins-Klein. I enrolled in her book writing course by the Book Midwife, and her process helped me write the most authentic book with my voice that I possibly could.

A massive thank-you to my husband, Sandeep Khatri, for always supporting my dreams and helping me turn my business and this book into a reality. His support has no limits. His love has no boundaries. He has this never-ending faith in my ability to guide my students and clients towards balanced health.

AUTHOR BIO

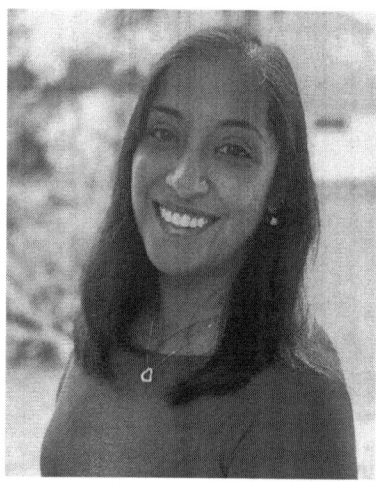

Varsha Khatri's approach to healing and living a healthy life is through the principles of Ayurveda, nutrition, health education, and yoga. She passionately believes that we make choices each day, and these decisions influence our health. Through her work, she shows passion and commitment to health promotion and disease prevention.

Over the years, her international experience in the field of holistic health has enabled her to work with patients to reach their health goals through the power of healing foods. Varsha founded her own health and wellness business, Illuminated Health, in 2012. She uses techniques from both Eastern and Western health practices. Her private practice involves integrating both the Western and the Ayurvedic approach to diet, nutrition, fitness, lifestyle, and spirituality. She also teaches yoga, provides nutrition consultations, and regularly runs health and well-being courses to help people achieve their health goals.

Varsha has a master's degree in holistic health education with an emphasis in holistic nutrition, as well as a bachelor's degree in physiology and health, with an emphasis in Maharishi Ayurveda. She is a registered senior yoga teacher. As a qualified nutritionist, Varsha specialises in working with children's health, digestive health, food allergies, and autoimmune conditions. She motivates and inspires her clients to work at a pace that is comfortable yet challenging while also educating them along the way so they continue to make healthier choices. Her approach is practical and recognises that each individual is different.

Originally from San Diego, California, Varsha now lives in Greater London with her husband and two kids, where she runs Illuminated Health. Varsha loves to spend time with her children and get them involved with many of her wellness activities, such as yoga and cooking. Aside from yoga and meditation, Varsha loves reading, going for walks, colouring, spending time outdoors, and crocheting. She and her husband like to live by example for their children by making healthy choices within their own family diet and lifestyle.

You can find out more about Varsha and all her work by visiting her website, www.illuminatedhealth.com. She can also be found on Facebook and Instagram: @illuminatedhealth. Varsha runs an online community group on Facebook: Healthy Living with Varsha which is open to anyone to join.

ENDNOTES

1   Nuttall, F. "Body Mass Index, Obesity, BMI, and Health: A Critical Review". 2015, April 7. https://www.ncbi.nlm.nih.gov/pmc/articles/PMC4890841.

2   "Health at Every Size", https://haescommunity.com.

3   Medline Plus. "Amino Acids". 2020, Nov 7. https://medlineplus.gov/ency/article/002222.htm

4   Arnarson, A. "Signs and Symptoms of Protein Deficiency". 2017, Oct 31. https://www.healthline.com/nutrition/protein-deficiency-symptoms#TOC_TITLE_HDR_9.

5   Harvard Health Publishing. "When It Comes to Protein, How Much Is Too Much?. 2020, March 30. https://www.health.harvard.edu/nutrition/when-it-comes-to-protein-how-much-is-too-much.

6   National Institute of General Medical Sciences. "Circadian Rhythms". 2020, Nov 8. https://www.nigms.nih.gov/education/fact-sheets/Pages/circadian-rhythms.aspx.

7   *Mosby's Dictionary of Medicine, Nursing, and Health Professions* 7th edition. St. Louis. Elsevier. 2006.

8   *Charaka Samhita*, Sutrasthan, 11.37

9   Pencavel, John. "The Productivity Of Working Hours", 2013, https://siepr.stanford.edu/sites/default/files/publications/FatiguepaperSIEPRcover_0.pdf.

10 Jeffrey Bland et al., *Clinical Nutrition: A Functional Approach* 2nd edition. Gig Harbor. The Institute for Functional Medicine. 2004.

11 The Endocrine Society. (2016, April 2). "Most People Cycle and Regain Weight, and Those Who Lose Most Are Most Likely to Keep It Off". *ScienceDaily*. www.sciencedaily.com/releases/2016/04/160402112741.htm

12 Hey, William T., et al. "Use of Body-Mind-Spirit Dimensions for the Development of a Wellness Behavior and Characteristic Inventory for College Students." *Health Promotion Practice*, vol. 7, no. 1, 2006, pp. 125–133. JSTOR, www.jstor.org/stable/26736351.

[13] Maharishi Ayurveda. "A Brief History of Maharishi Ayurveda". 2020, Nov 9. https://www.maharishi.co.uk/maharishi-ayurveda-history

[14] Sharma, Hari and Clark, Christopher. *Contemporary Ayurveda.* Independence Square West. Churchill Livingstone. 2002.

[15] Narayanaswamy, V. "Origin and Development of Ayurveda. (A Brief History)". https://www.ncbi.nlm.nih.gov/pmc/articles/PMC3336651/pdf/ASL-1-1.pdf 1981

[16] Yogi, M. (2007, April 12). *Lesson 4: Improving Digestion - Consciousness Based Approach.* Lecture presented at MIU, Fairfield. Course Diet, Digestion, Nutrition. Taught by Janet Kernis.

[17] Charaka Samhita, Vimanasthan, 1.5

[18] Morehead, P. (2006, October). Course on *Prevention.* Quote shared from Charak Samhita during course.

[19] Mayo Clinic. "Supplements: Nutrition in a Pill". 2020, Nov 17. https://www.mayoclinic.org/healthy-lifestyle/nutrition-and-healthy-eating/in-depth/supplements/art-20044894

[20] Pacheco, D. "Why Electronics Affect Sleep". 2020, Nov 6. https://www.sleepfoundation.org/articles/why-electronics-may-stimulate-you-bed

[21] Sushrut Samhita, Sutrasthan, 15.41

[22] Centers for Disease Control and Prevention. "What Are the Risk Factors for Lung Cancer?" 2020, Nov 16. https://www.cdc.gov/cancer/lung/basic_info/risk_factors.htm

[23] National Institutes of Health. "Health Consequences for Drug Misuse" 2020, June. https://www.drugabuse.gov/drug-topics/health-consequences-drug-misuse/mental-health-effects

[24] National Institute on Alcohol Abuse and Alcoholism. "The Epidemiology of Alcoholic Liver Disease". Alcohol Research & Health. 2003. Robert E. Mann, Ph.D., et.al. https://pubs.niaaa.nih.gov/publications/arh27-3/209-219.htm

[25] "Your Guide to Food Intolerance Testing". https://www.yorktest.com/buyers-guide/

[26] NHS. "Constipation". 2020, Nov 16. https://www.nhs.uk/conditions/constipation/

[27] Madhav Nidan Samhita, VI 5, 10-12

[28] Tolle, Eckhart. *Power of Now: A Guide to Spiritual Enlightenment.* New World Library. 2004.

[29] "#100happydays" 2020, Nov 16. https://100happydays.com

[30] Simioni, C., Zauli, G., Martelli, A. M., Vitale, M., Sacchetti, G., Gonelli, A., & Neri, L. M. (2018). "Oxidative Stress: Role of Physical Exercise and

Antioxidant Nutraceuticals in Adulthood and Aging". *Oncotarget, 9*(24), 17181–17198. https://doi.org/10.18632/oncotarget.24729

31 Jeffrey Bland et al., *Clinical Nutrition: A Functional Approach* 2nd edition. Gig Harbor. The Institute for Functional Medicine. 2004.

32 Dr Murray, Michael., Dr. Pizzorno, Joseph. Pizzorno, Lara. *The Encyclopaedia of Healing Foods.* London. Piatkus. 2013

33 Dr Murray, Michael., Dr. Pizzorno, Joseph. Pizzorno, Lara. *The Encyclopaedia of Healing Foods.* London. Piatkus. 2013

34 Minich, Deanna. *The Rainbow Diet Color Wheel.* 2020, Nov 16. https://www.deannaminich.com/downloads/

35 Brown, Peter. "Increase Ojas to Promote Heart Health" 2013, Dec 2. https://www.maharishi.co.uk/blog/increase-ojas-promote-heart-health/

36 Takahashi, Y., Kipnis, D. M., & Daughaday, W. H. (1968). "Growth Hormone Secretion during Sleep". *The Journal of Clinical Investigation*, 47(9), 2079–2090. https://doi.org/10.1172/JCI105893

37 Mayo Clinic. *Stress relief from laughter? It's no joke.* 2019, April 05. https://www.mayoclinic.org/healthy-lifestyle/stress-management/in-depth/stress-relief/art-20044456

38 Kubu, Cynthia PhD and Machado, Andre MD. "The Science Is Clear, Why Multitasking Doesn't Work". 2020, Nov 17. https://health.clevelandclinic.org/science-clear-multitasking-doesnt-work/

39 American Psychological Association. "Mindfulness meditation: A research-proven way to reduce stress." 2019, Oct 30.

40 Drug Science. "Caffeine". 2020, Nov 17. https://drugscience.org.uk/drug-information/caffeine/#368407893977959

41 Madell, Robin. "Exercise as Stress Relief". 2020, March 26. https://www.healthline.com/health/heart-disease/exercise-stress-relief#How-Much-Exercise-Do-You-Need?

42 Mayo Clinic. "Walking: Trim Your Waistline, Improve Your Health". 2019, Feb 27. https://www.mayoclinic.org/healthy-lifestyle/fitness/in-depth/walking/art-20046261

Printed and bound by CPI Group (UK) Ltd, Croydon, CR0 4YY